Ginger for Health

100 Amazing and Unexpected Uses for Ginger

Britt Brandon, CFNS, CPT

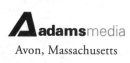

Avon, Massachusetts

DEDICATION

This book is dedicated to the loves of my life: Jimmy, Lilly, Lonni, and JD.

Published by
Adams Media, a division of F+W Media, Inc.
57 Littlefield Street, Avon, MA 02322. U.S.A.
www.adamsmedia.com

ISBN 10: 1-4405-9143-1
ISBN 13: 978-1-4405-9143-3
eISBN 10: 1-4405-9144-X
eISBN 13: 978-1-4405-9144-0

Printed in the United States of America.

10 9 8 7 6 5 4

Library of Congress Cataloging-in-Publication Data

Brandon, Britt.
  Ginger for health / Britt Brandon.
    pages cm
  Includes index.
  ISBN 978-1-4405-9143-3 (pb) -- ISBN 1-4405-9143-1
(pb) -- ISBN 978-1-4405-9144-0 (ebook) -- ISBN 1-4405-
9144-X (ebook)
  1. Ginger--Therapeutic use. I. Title.
  RM666.G488B73 2015
  615.3'2439--dc23
                              2015019029

Many of the designations used by manufacturers and sell-
ers to distinguish their products are claimed as trademarks.
Where those designations appear in this book and F+W
Media, Inc. was aware of a trademark claim, the designations
have been printed with initial capital letters.

The various uses of ginger as a health aid are based on
tradition, scientific theories, or limited research. They
often have not been thoroughly tested in humans, and
safety and effectiveness have not yet been proven in clini-
cal trials. Some of the conditions for which ginger can be
used as a treatment or remedy are potentially serious, and
should be evaluated by a qualified health-care provider.

This book is intended as general information only, and
should not be used to diagnose or treat any health condition.
In light of the complex, individual, and specific nature of
health problems, this book is not intended to replace professional medical advice. The ideas, procedures, and suggestions
in this book are intended to supplement, not replace, the advice of a trained medical professional. Consult your physician before adopting any of the suggestions in this book, as
well as about any condition that may require diagnosis or
medical attention. The author and publisher disclaim any li-
ability arising directly or indirectly from the use of this book.

Cover design by Michelle Roy Kelly.
Cover image © iStockphoto.com/AlexRaths.

*This book is available at quantity discounts for bulk purchases.
For information, please call 1-800-289-0963.*

CONTENTS

PART II: BEAUTY   85

Chapter 3: Skin Care   86

Chapter 4: Hair Care   108

INTRODUCTION

Do you want to lose weight? Alleviate allergy symptoms? Moisturize your skin? Treat dandruff?

What if I told you that there was a special root that had been used for thousands of years to effectively treat these and other issues, and that this unique wonder-root may very well be in your refrigerator right now?

This powerful superfood that could possibly change your life for the better is none other than ginger, an age-old root that not only improves healing, promotes vitality, and improves the body's functioning, but is also versatile enough to include in a variety of dishes that range from sweet to salty, and spicy to subtle. And to add to the world-wide reputation of this amazing superfood's healing capabilities are the new scientific studies done over the past decades that have shown that this herb contains powerful unique vitamins, minerals, antioxidants, and compounds that literally work wonders in every area of your health and life!

While traditional Chinese and Ayurvedic medicines have relied on the ginger root for healing common ailments for thousands of years, this herb has only recently made an astounding reputation for itself as a superfood that is capable of not only healing minor illnesses, but safeguarding and improving overall health as well. With a growing percentage of the population turning to natural treatment methods as opposed to modern medicines, the ginger root and its natural healing capabilities have been thrust into the spotlight, commanding the attention of natural healers and those seeking natural health-improving dietary elements. And, in fact, recent scientific studies and in-depth research have now identified the powerful compounds in the ginger root that can improve the body's natural processes and minimize a number of common conditions experienced by people of all ages, genders, and walks of life. From diabetes to heart disease, to colds and flus, to cancers, the natural healing power of ginger has shown to be quite extraordinary.

And, in addition to its healing powers, ginger also makes the perfect addition to a natural beauty regimen. With a number of simple, yet effective, applications for the skin and hair that utilize ginger and all of its healing nutrients and phytochemicals, anyone can improve the appearance and health of their skin and hair. Beauty-boosting benefits from the same nutrients, antioxidants, anti-inflammatory compounds, oils, and enzymes that promote internal health throughout the body can naturally improve the health of your body—inside *and* out!

On the following pages, you'll find 100 benefits and ways to use this delightful ingredient that can not only add spice to your culinary creations, but improve your health, beauty, and life in astounding ways!

GINGER'S MANY HEALTH BENEFITS

What Is Ginger?

Before we start talking about ginger's benefits, let's talk about what ginger actually is. You may be surprised to learn that the ginger you know and love is actually the root of a beautiful red, white, or yellow and green flowering plant that belongs to the zingiberaceae family, to which other well-known spices like turmeric and cardamom also belong. The ginger root is a knotted, tubular-shaped root with a light yellow, white, or red flesh that is covered with a silvery exterior coating. The name "ginger" originated more than 3,000 years ago in early Sanskrit writings that referred to the root as *gingivere*, meaning "horn root," which describes the root's unique appearance.

How to Select, Store, and Prepare Ginger

Depending upon how young the plant is at the time of harvest, the ginger root's exterior coating can be thick or thin. The thickness of this shiny coating is an indication of the root's nutritional content, as ginger roots that are allowed to age to a year or more before harvest have been shown to provide beneficial oils in a greater concentration than the roots of plants harvested earlier. When selecting ginger, you want to make sure you're buying fresh varieties of the later-harvested, more beneficial roots, so look for roots that are firm and heavy for their size, with a smooth exterior and a spicy fragrance that signifies a rich concentration of nutrients. Avoid roots that feel light for their size or have wrinkled flesh, as these roots were either selected too early or are too aged, either situation yielding a ginger root with far fewer nutrients and phytochemicals.

When storing ginger, the roots can be wrapped in paper towels, placed in a sealable plastic bag, and stored in the refrigerator for up to three weeks or the freezer for up to two months. Dried ginger can be stored in an airtight container set in a cool, dark space for up to six months. Pickled ginger can be stored in an airtight container in the refrigerator for up to three months. To prepare ginger, simply peel the exterior coating with a peeler, and mince, slice, shred, or grate as needed. A helpful tip when slicing ginger is to slice the root perpendicular to the fibers; this will help minimize the stringiness of the fibers within the slices.

The History of Ginger

The ginger plant has been used around the world by countless cultures and civilizations, but it originated in China. But while the plant is indigenous to Asia, it has spread throughout the world over the past 5,000 years. Ginger has been a well-known staple of cultures and civilizations around the world, as seen in documents that date back thousands of years, mentioned by Greek physician and pharmacist Pedanius Dioscorides; seen in the writings of the Chinese philosopher Confucius; found in the Arabic collection of folk tales, *One Thousand and One Nights*; and even referred to in the Koran. The plant's popularity spread from China to the Maluku Islands (called the Spice Islands); around A.D. 100 ginger quickly took hold in West Africa, the Caribbean, and then Europe. While these various cultures used the ginger root for similar purposes, the unique uses that were discovered for the special spice increased and improved over time. Once thought to be an effective reliever of stomach issues and common colds, the ginger root evolved into an aphrodisiac, a sore throat soother, a blood cleanser, a wound healer, and much more! Over the course of time, this root has been used in every form imaginable: powdered, crushed, minced, sliced, and pickled. Even when candied, this root contains natural compounds that promote health in every form. Today, the scientific exploration of the ginger root's compounds still continues to unveil new and exciting capabilities and uses.

Over time, as the rapid growth of the harvesting and exportation of ginger proved successful and lucrative, the race to become the leader in the ginger industry narrowed to just two countries: China and India. While China held the lead for a number of years, India currently holds the top spot for ginger production and exportation with an astounding 703,000 tons of ginger produced in 2012. 2.1 million tons of ginger are produced annually worldwide, giving the consumers of the glorious root peace of mind in knowing that their favorite flavor and health enhancer will be available year-round for the foreseeable future.

The Special Benefits of Ginger

The ginger root possesses natural oils, amino acids, vitamins, minerals, fatty acids, and phytochemicals that combine to provide healing properties for almost every area of the body. Phytochemicals are naturally occurring plant compounds that boost the healthy functioning of cells, tissues, organs, and systems. These compounds include antioxidants, anti-inflammatory agents, analgesics, and a wide variety of protective, preventative, and health-promoting derivatives that help support the natural functions of the body. The powerful oils contained within the flesh of the ginger root are varieties of gingerol, paradol, shogaol, and gingerdione, which not only help combat germs, bacteria, and viruses, but also help stimulate the senses, improve energy, increase metabolic functioning, and cleanse the blood.

We'll go into more depth on the benefits of ginger throughout the book, but here is some basic info on ginger's powerful benefits.

Amino Acids

The amino acids provided by the ginger root include each of the ten essential amino acids we must consume through food because, unlike the non-essential amino acids, the human body does not naturally produce them. The amino acids found in ginger root are:

- *Arginine*: helps to eliminate toxins from the body; aids in the production of the energy compound creatine, which is required in the process of energy production and by the muscles for movement; acts as a natural vasodilator, naturally opening and expanding the blood vessels for improved blood flow; and has been found to reduce chest pain, the risk of heart failure, and headaches.
- *Histidine*: improves the body's immune system functioning by aiding in the fight against pathogens, is necessary for the formation of blood cells, and directly improves a variety of arthritis symptoms as well as high blood pressure.

- *Isoleucine*: promotes muscle recovery after exercise; regulates blood sugar; aids proper blood clotting and in the formation of hemoglobin, the oxygen-transporting blood protein; and helps the body fight infection.
- *Leucine*: the strongest of the branched-chain amino acids (leucine, isoleucine, and valine combine to create the branched-chain amino acid group, referred to as BCAA), essential for energy production and muscle growth; helps to regulate blood sugar; aids in the repair of muscles, tissue, and bone; helps with wound healing; and elevates energy levels.
- *Lysine*: necessary for calcium absorption, for the conversion of fat to energy, and for the production of hormones, antibodies, collagen, tissue, and muscle; maintains blood cell health; and promotes new muscle growth.
- *Methionine*: assists in the breakdown and uses of fats in the bloodstream; aids in detoxification; promotes proper digestion; required for creatine production; improves energy production; and aids muscle maintenance and growth.
- *Phenylalanine*: stimulates the nervous system; elevates and regulates mood; aids in memory processes; and increases the production of epinephrine and dopamine, two neurotransmitters produced in the brain that directly affect cognitive processes.
- *Threonine*: used to form collagen and elastin, two essential protein fibers used to make up the composition of the skin; promotes bone and tissue health, and healthy liver functioning; maintains protein balance throughout the body; aids in production of antibodies; and improves immunity by promoting the healthy functioning of the thymus, as well as proper protein and mineral absorption and use.
- *Tryptophan*: required for proper B-vitamin absorption and use, and for the production of serotonin and other mood-related neurotransmitters; stabilizes mood; promotes sleep; improves immunity; and is necessary for the production of collagen, enamel, and elastin, all of which are directly related to the health of the internal systems' functioning and the appearance of the external organs like hair, skin, and nails.
- *Valine*: aids in the repair and growth of muscles; maintains proper nitrogen balance in the body for optimal protein synthesis and use; and preserves the body's natural stores of glucose for improved energy production.

Vitamins

The vitamins obtained through food help support every organ, system, and function in the body. With each vitamin delivering energy, improving immunity, protecting cell health, and maintaining proper metabolic functioning, it's easy to see why these nutrients are essential, and why avoiding a deficiency of any vitamin is crucial to maintaining overall health. Ginger provides a number of essential vitamins, and also contains natural oils and enzymes that improve the body's ability to absorb, process, and utilize vitamins for maximum benefits. The vitamins provided by ginger include:

- *Vitamin A*: essential for vision health and prevention of cataracts; helps with the formation of hormones and the maintenance of teeth, tissue, and cell membrane health; works to maintain healthy hair production; and prevents oxidative activity in cells that can destroy cell health or transform cells to cancerous copies of themselves.
- *B Vitamins*: essential energy-boosting vitamins that contribute to muscle health, assist in protein synthesis, and assist in the metabolism of all nutrients throughout the body. Certain B vitamins can also prevent neural tube defects in fetuses, are required for the formation of blood cells and DNA, and promote healthy brain functioning.
- *Vitamin C*: antiviral agent and powerful antioxidant that prevents oxidative and free radical activity in cells that can turn healthy cells to damaged cells responsible for the development of serious illnesses and diseases like cancer; required for the absorption and use of iron, calcium, and folate; helps build and maintain healthy bones, teeth, gums, and blood vessels; assists in wound and bruise healing; and fights infection. This vitamin cannot be stored in the body, and must therefore be regularly consumed in appropriate amounts.

Minerals

Minerals are the essential nutrients obtained from foods that help support the structures and processes in the body. Contributing to the health of the bones, teeth, hair, skin, and nails, minerals also maintain the health of the heart, brain, and digestive system by cleansing the blood, improving nerve health, boosting immunity, and upholding the heart and cardiovascular system's strength. The minerals provided by ginger include:

- *Calcium*: aids in the cell's absorption of nutrients, required for muscle contractions that allow us to move, jump, and exercise, and also pump blood throughout the heart and body; promotes proper blood clotting; supports bone health; essential for proper nerve functioning and communication; required for insulin production and secretion; improves immune system functioning by playing a role in the enzymatic reactions of T-cells in the immune system; involved in the production of white blood cells; and promotes healthy sleep.
- *Iron*: improves immune system functioning; promotes brain functioning, mental clarity, and energy; fights fatigue; and increases the body's absorption of vitamin C.
- *Magnesium*: supports bone health; required for the formation of cells; involved in protein absorption, production, and use; assists in the body's absorption and use of B vitamins; promotes energy production, insulin production, and secretion; improves nervous system functioning; involved in muscle repair; and assists in the absorption of calcium, vitamin C, and potassium.
- *Manganese*: required for the enzymatic reactions that take place in the body for hormone production, energy use, and a number of metabolic processes; regulates blood sugar levels; improves metabolic functioning; and is essential for the production of thyroid hormones.
- *Phosphorous*: combines with calcium to promote the healthy formation of bones and teeth; and promotes healthy nervous system functioning.
- *Potassium*: promotes proper growth of the body's bones, muscles, and tissues; maintains healthy fluid balance within cells; prevents muscle cramping; promotes healthy kidney functioning and cardiovascular system functioning (specifically required for the maintenance of a healthy heartbeat); and supports the respiratory system by strengthening the lungs and improving the processes related to breathing and processing oxygen.

- *Sodium*: regulates blood pressure; regulates fluid balance within cells and throughout the body; and is required for the healthy functioning of the nerves and muscles.
- *Zinc*: required for the metabolism of proteins and carbohydrates; promotes healthy immune system functioning; and supports wound healing and eye health.

Overall Health

Through the use of quality nutrients found in natural foods, the body benefits immensely. With rich provisions of essential nutrients like amino acids, vitamins, and minerals, along with oils and enzymes that help the body process those essential nutrients, ginger is the perfect addition to a daily diet or beauty routine for maximum benefits to the body, inside and out. Helping to maintain the health of the body's cells, tissues, organs, and systems, this sweet spice is a splendid way to provide your body with prevention, protection, and health-boosting nutrition that improves and maintains optimal overall health.

PART I

HEALTH

Chapter 1
NUTRITION

Without question, quality nutrition is essential to achieve and maintain optimal health. After all, the protein, carbohydrates, fats, vitamins, minerals, and amino acids provided to your body through food are what allow the body to function. When the body is depleted or deprived of the nutrients it requires for its basic functions and processes, the results can be life-altering or even life-threatening. But, when the body is supplied with an abundance of nutrients that promote the functioning of every system throughout the body, the results can be extraordinary!

If you could add an element to your daily diet that would not just enable your body to simply function, but actually encourage it to thrive, wouldn't you do it? What if that single dietary addition could improve every aspect of your life from mental functioning and physical performance, to improved mood balance to increased energy, to even increased weight loss and reduced toxicity? Most people would jump at the chance to experience all there is to offer. The great news is that this addition exists, and is none other than ginger!

To gain the benefits detailed throughout this chapter, you need to consume 2–4 tablespoons (or the dried equivalent) of fresh ginger per day. A 1" piece of ginger will produce approximately 1 tablespoon of freshly grated ginger, which is equivalent to 1 teaspoon of ground ginger. How you choose to ingest your ginger is up to you! Add it to a smoothie, use it to spice up soups and salads, or make some magic with your favorite meals. As long as you get the ginger you need, you'll be on the road to better nutrition before you know it. So let's take a look at how you can use ginger to move from just functioning to thriving!

1. CONTRIBUTES B VITAMINS

The B vitamins are essential, whether you hope to improve your immunity, increase your metabolic functioning, or maintain heart, nerve, and muscle health. Ginger contributes the six B vitamins found in plant foods, and improves the processes responsible for the absorption and utilization of those vitamins, which increases their effectiveness. With the addition of ginger to your diet, you may begin to experience more of the benefits that result from having essential B vitamins in the diet, which include:

- *Vitamin B_1* (thiamin): converts carbohydrates from food to energy; maintains health of skin, hair, and nails; promotes healthy functioning of the cardiovascular and nervous system; maintains heart health; and fights fatigue.
- *Vitamin B_2* (riboflavin): promotes healthy growth of bones, muscles, and tissues; maintains reproductive health; aids the body's process of converting carbohydrates to energy; and is essential for red blood cell production.
- *Vitamin B_3* (niacin): promotes healthy digestion; essential for nervous system functioning; promotes mental clarity; improves metabolic functioning; involved in the process of converting food to usable energy; and promotes the health of skin, nails, and hair.

- *Vitamin B_5* (pantothenic acid): essential for metabolic functioning; involved in hormone production; and promotes proper levels of good cholesterol (HDL) in the blood.
- *Vitamin B_6* (pyridoxine): improves immune and nervous system functioning; necessary for the production of essential antibodies used to support immune system functioning and fend off illness and disease; involved in blood cell production; and required for the enzymatic reactions involved in the body's processes of absorbing, storing, and utilizing protein.
- *Vitamin B_9* (folate): occurs naturally in foods (as opposed to folic acid that is chemically formulated); prevents neural tube defects in fetuses; required for the formation of blood cells and DNA; promotes healthy brain functioning.

These B vitamins are energy-boosting nutrients the body needs to fight fatigue, and the benefits don't stop there! Helping to keep the brain, heart, bones, and nerves healthy and ensuring their healthy functioning and growth, the B's are essential for achieving and maintaining optimal overall health.

2. ADDS AMINO ACIDS TO YOUR DIET

The amino acids are powerful "building blocks" used by the body to perform processes that are needed for everything from basic functioning to the maintenance of physical, mental, and emotional well-being. Our bodies require essential amino acids for everything from natural regulation of blood sugar, hormone levels, metabolism, energy production, and even the maintenance of a healthy heartbeat. Without the proper amounts of amino acids, every process, system, and organ can be adversely affected. There are two types of amino acids: essential and non-essential. The difference between the essential and non-essential amino acids is their origin; while the body can manufacture non-essential amino acids ("non-essential" meaning quite literally, that they are not essential because the body can create them naturally), the "essential" amino acids must be obtained through natural foods to promote and maintain your body's optimal functioning.

While there are many foods you can eat that will provide you with essential amino acids, the ones most popular for being amino acid-rich are animal products such as meat and dairy foods. Plants are also packed full of amino acids, and ginger is one of them that not only adds amino acids to your diet,

but also helps your body process and use those amino acids in the most beneficial ways possible. Because of the vitamins, minerals, and naturally occurring oils and phytochemicals in ginger, the absorption and utilization of the essential amino acids improves while the manufacturing and processing of the body's own non-essential amino acids also improves! With the combination of increased vitamins and minerals, additional essential amino acids added to the diet, and improved production and processing of the non-essential amino acids, the body's benefits from ginger can be quite astounding!

AWAY WITH ANTIBIOTICS

Antibiotics are prescribed with the intention of killing bacterial infections in the body, but these powerful medications do not discriminate. Killing off all bacteria, good and bad, antibiotics can devastate the normal balance of healthy bacteria in the blood and body that are responsible for everything from aiding digestion to keeping yeast overgrowth under control. By opting for natural bacterial remedies like ginger, you can maintain healthy levels of beneficial bacteria while fending off bad bacteria, microbes, and viruses.

3. IMPROVES CALCIUM ABSORPTION

Calcium is a widely recognized mineral that is most commonly thought of in terms of its maintenance of bone health. And in fact, a deficiency in this essential mineral can actually cause the body to detract it from where it is stored in the bones and teeth, making those sources susceptible to deterioration. But, while calcium is absolutely essential for the formation and maintenance of strong and healthy bones and teeth, it's also necessary for a number of functions throughout the body that (according to some) far surpass the importance of bone health.

Required for the formation of healthy DNA and RNA, the need for calcium begins at the moment of conception. Throughout the gestation of a fetus, calcium is required for almost every process, enzymatic reaction, and development of every organ and system throughout the body. After birth and throughout life, this essential mineral is used by the circulatory, nervous, skeletal, muscular, immune, digestive, and reproductive systems.

Fortunately, the calcium in ginger helps keep these systems working at full speed, and it also provides support to the body's calcium stores, by processing and utilizing this mineral in a number of ways that help to improve the body's functioning and contribute to overall health. And because ginger is full of vitamin C, vitamin E, and magnesium, which have been shown to improve the body's natural process of eliminating sodium, improve the digestive process, and maintain proper protein metabolism, it is able to make sure the body has optimal calcium stores, which keep it functioning at its healthiest!

4. IMPROVES IRON ABSORPTION

Iron is another essential mineral that is responsible for the healthy functioning of almost every system and process throughout the body. It works to form hemoglobin in the blood, deliver oxygen throughout the body, improve the production of red and white blood cells, and maintain the immune system to help reduce the risk of illness and infection. If you have an insufficient amount of iron in your body, you'll quickly feel the effects: drowsiness and fatigue, "foggy" mental processing, reduced immune system functioning, and frequent muscle fatigue. A diet rich in leafy greens can improve the body's stores of iron, but this is sometimes simply not enough. Fortunately, ginger is not only able to provide the body with small amounts of iron, but it is—more importantly—able to help the body extract and utilize iron more efficiently through its provisions of vitamin C and a number of supportive, naturally occurring oils. In a 2012 study led by Dr. Rashmi Kulkarni and featured in *The Indian Journal of Traditional Knowledge*, 62 participants between the ages of 18 and 55 suffering from iron deficiency were given either ginger or a placebo every day. Following analysis of the iron levels of the participants, the researchers concluded that ginger assisted in iron absorption and "was found to be beneficial as a support in the therapy of anemia." So, with the additional benefits that can result from its consumption, coupled with the scientific proof of its positive effects on iron absorption, ginger is an important addition to the diet of every person in need of improved or optimal iron functioning.

5. REDUCES BAD CHOLESTEROL

Most people hear "cholesterol" and automatically assume that it is a danger to the body. This isn't necessarily true, so it's important to clarify that cholesterol is actually needed by the body in a number of functions and processes, and only becomes a danger when there are excessive levels of the "bad" kind of cholesterol. The body naturally processes the cholesterol consumed from food and produced by the body, and uses it for a number of processes required by cells, organs, and systems. Because the body isn't able to dissolve cholesterol in the blood, the cholesterol is used throughout the body as needed, and the excess is excreted.

The issues concerning cholesterol come into play when the bad cholesterol, commonly referred to as "low-density lipoproteins" (or LDL) cholesterol, contributes to the creation of a plaque that is formed within the blood and deposited on the walls of arteries. These deposits make the arteries stiff and less flexible or create blockages, minimizing blood flow to and from the heart and throughout the body, leading to a condition known as atherosclerosis, which can result in heart attacks and strokes. Because there are usually no symptoms to indicate the buildup of this bad cholesterol, it is imperative to have your blood cholesterol levels checked regularly.

While many people turn to prescription medications to reduce their LDL cholesterol levels, research shows that specific foods—including ginger!—can improve these levels naturally. A 2008 study conducted by Dr. Alizadeh-Navaei and published in the *Saudi Medical Journal* showed that "ginger has a significant lipid-lowering effect compared to the placebo," while a 2000 Israeli study concluded that "dietary consumption of ginger extract significantly attenuates the . . . LDL cholesterol levels." With the improvements that occur throughout the body as a result of introducing ginger to the diet, the reduction of LDL cholesterol levels is just one more way that ginger can not only improve your health, but also improve the quality *and* the length of your life!

6. IMPROVES GOOD CHOLESTEROL

While ginger can reduce the amount of "bad cholesterol" in your body, it can also boost the amount of "good cholesterol" (also known as "high-density lipoproteins" or HDL) that your body needs to function properly. As we discussed in the previous entry, cholesterol is required for the maintenance of cell walls and membranes, the production of hormones, processing of vitamin D, and the metabolism of fats, and is necessary for the body to function optimally. Ideally, the body is able to use the cholesterol obtained from food and produced naturally within the body for the functions and processes in which it's required, but efficiently excrete the excess without having deposits of the cholesterol left behind.

With a focus on diet becoming the leading recommendation for improving cholesterol and safeguarding heart health, it's no wonder that ginger has become a superfood in this specific area. In addition to its ability to reduce the "bad cholesterol" levels of the blood, ginger improves the metabolic, cardiovascular, and hormone-producing functions of the body, which in turn helps improve the processing, utilization, and excretion of cholesterol. With the added benefits that result from ginger's support of proper circulation and blood-cleansing properties, this root is able to encourage the transport and filtering of cholesterol throughout the body for use or removal. Ginger's detoxifying properties also encourage the liver's proper processing of cholesterol. Through ginger's support of these systems and functions, the body is able to better regulate cholesterol levels and use the HDL cholesterol for the body's optimal functioning and improved health.

7. REGULATES INSULIN LEVELS

Insulin, a naturally occurring hormone produced by the pancreas, is the body's natural blood-sugar regulation tool that is needed to maintain optimal sources of energy for the cells. When you consume food, the sugars in those foods tell your body's pancreas to release insulin; the insulin then allows the sugar (which is converted to blood glucose) to enter the cells, which then use the glucose for energy. Excess glucose is stored in the liver and released as the body needs it for processes relating to hormonal balance, blood sugar levels, or enzymatic reactions that are necessary for insulin release or use, or to maintain normal blood glucose levels. With insulin sensitivity, Type I diabetes, or Type II diabetes, the lack of proper insulin functions can result in major health issues such as fatigue, poor healing ability, or amputation resulting from poor blood flow and delivery.

While medications for insulin-related conditions are commonly prescribed, many physicians and patients are searching for natural treatment alternatives that minimize the risk of side effects and promote the overall functioning and health of the body. Ginger has come to the forefront of these natural treatment methods, and for a great reason. In three major scientific studies that have been performed since 2005, it has been determined that "ginger extract reduced blood levels of insulin by 10 percent and blood sugar by 35 percent," "ginger extract helps increase cells' absorption of glucose independent of insulin," and that "ginger recipients experienced improved insulin sensitivity, lower levels of insulin, and significantly lower levels of LDL cholesterol and triglycerides." Giving hope to the millions of physicians, researchers, and patients who deal with diabetes on a daily basis, ginger is one of the natural healing alternatives that in future years may make this condition, and many others, a thing of the past.

TALK TO YOUR DOCTOR

While ginger's abilities in dealing with diabetes are nothing short of astounding, it should be made clear that changes to one's treatment plan, or introducing ginger to the diet of a diabetic, should always be discussed at length with a physician first. With the use of ginger's natural healing powers, the life of a diabetic can improve dramatically, but it should never be considered an option that would displace insulin treatments altogether without complete supervision and approval by a physician.

8. IMPROVES METABOLIC FUNCTIONING

The term "metabolism" refers to the functioning of all of the body's cells in a variety of processes that are classified as either catabolic (breaks down elements into usable forms of energy) or anabolic (creates compounds that are needed by the cells). In order to perform basic daily functions, the body has a resting metabolic rate that provides the energy needed to think, breathe, digest, pump blood, and even blink your eyes.

Physical demands beyond this rate (such as exercise) require more energy, which puts increased demands on the metabolism. Basically, metabolism is a constantly running machine that can run well or poorly, depending upon a number of factors ranging from diet and exercise, to a person's quality of health, to the body's ability to function properly for optimal metabolic support.

As ginger offers a helping hand to the specific supporting endocrine, nervous, cardiovascular, and digestive systems and the precise processes like hormone production and regulation, and the synthesis, storage, and use of carbohydrates, proteins, and fats that directly support the optimal functioning of the metabolism, it's no surprise that the spicy root has been shown to remarkably improve metabolic functioning. Not only does ginger provide support to the very systems and processes that indirectly affect the metabolism, it also enhances areas that have direct effects on metabolic performance, such as the increased calorie burn, energy production, and alertness that result from the thermogenic effect produced by the natural spiciness of ginger.

By revving the metabolic engine and promoting the proper functioning of the metabolism, ginger can actually improve the most basic cellular functioning in the body (improving all of the body's systems with which those cells communicate), but can also help improve the energy, focus, and fire that every body needs in order to be its healthiest throughout life!

RESTING METABOLIC RATE

If you're interested in calculating your resting metabolic rate, use these equations: For men: 66 + (6.23 × weight in lbs.) + (12.7 × height in inches) − (6.8 × age in years) = RMR. For women: 655 + (4.35 × weight in lbs.) + (4.7 × height in inches) − (4.7 × age in years) = RMR.

9. REDUCES SUGAR CRAVINGS

Sugar cravings can easily be described as strong (almost undeniable) urges to consume sugar. But what causes these widely recognized urges? Excessive stress, digestive troubles, hormone fluctuation, inadequate nutrient absorption, actual hunger, fatigue, low blood sugar levels, and even boredom or lack of focus can all be contributing factors to these sugar cravings. Note that these symptoms and the subsequent cravings can stem from physiological responses to a serious system malfunctioning rather than a "lack of willpower."

Regardless of what the source of your cravings may be, it's no surprise that ginger can help. With micronutrients, system-correcting benefits, and health-promoting properties, ginger is able to specifically target and improve the main sources of sugar cravings. Hormonal imbalances, blood sugar fluctuations, irregular digestion, mood and focus, and even sleep quality can all be improved or aided in adjustment with the consumption of ginger. With its unique enzymes that assist in hormonal imbalance correction, fiber for blood sugar regulation, oils and nutrients that improve digestion, antioxidants that assist in cognitive functioning, and analgesics and dopamine-improving enzymes, ginger helps all of these areas naturally. With the added benefits of improved metabolism, mental functioning, and optimal overall health, ginger may be the answer to your sugar cravings and so much more!

10. PROMOTES WEIGHT LOSS

The efficient way to achieve sustainable weight loss is through a collaboration of lifestyle changes that improve health and provide the body with the tools that it needs. These tools for weight loss aren't focused on one specific area of life (or even on one specific area of the body), but are rather a series of keys that lead to improved overall health. When combined, these keys gradually contribute to the loss of fat, the increase of muscle, and a new, improved lifestyle that is able to continue and sustain weight loss successfully. Some of the most important keys are:

- A diet focused on nutrient-dense natural foods
- A diet free of excessive sugar, sodium, and unhealthy fats
- An active lifestyle that promotes calorie burn
- An active exercise regimen that promotes muscle building and maintenance
- A lifestyle that promotes healthy sleep habits and reduction of stress
- A focus on promoting healthy hormone balance

Ginger can help you use any of these keys to unlock the door to weight loss!

Ginger begins the process of weight loss by enhancing the body's absorption of essential vitamins and minerals, helping to ensure the body has ample amounts of the very nutrients it needs to thrive (many that may have been missing in a diet contributing to weight gain). Also, through its natural provisions of metabolism-stimulating "spice," ginger has shown to be an effective aid in minimizing cravings for unhealthy foods laden with sugars, sodium, and unhealthy fats, while also increasing the metabolism's rate of functioning and contributing to energy levels (which always help with increased activity!), further contributing to an increased calorie burn. And, with its ability to regulate hormones that can directly affect stress, sleep, focus, and energy production (all needed to maintain a healthy weight), ginger can provide the support necessary to all of the body's systems simply, naturally, and deliciously!

11. PROVIDES PRE-WORKOUT ENERGY

While there are a countless number of pre-workout drinks on the market catering to the "needs" of those trying to care for their body with exercise and adequate nutrition, these marketed pre-workout drinks are filled with excessive sugars, unnecessary additives, preservatives, caffeine, and synthetic stimulants. Fortunately, with a simple, ginger-filled homemade concoction, you can enjoy the perfect pre-workout energy drink that's packed with everything your body needs to embark on a workout with sustained energy.

With the addition of just 1 tablespoon of grated ginger, the absorption of essential minerals that act as electrolytes (calcium, potassium, and magnesium) improves the muscles' endurance and recovery, while the added B vitamins promote energy. The unique compounds of ginger add the "spice" that improves metabolic functioning and calorie burn. The potassium-rich banana and the antioxidant-rich, naturally caffeinated green tea increase energy while also promoting cell health, and the natural sugars of the honey (when combined with the ginger) improve sustained energy levels and allow for a slow release of the sugars into the bloodstream. This drink also delivers essential nutrients throughout the body to ensure the muscles and all of the body's systems reap maximum benefits!

TO MAKE 1½ CUPS OF THIS ENERGIZING ELIXIR, COMBINE:

1 cup cooled green tea

1 banana, peeled and frozen

1 teaspoon raw organic honey

1 tablespoon grated ginger

Combine all ingredients in a blender and blend on high until all ingredients are completely emulsified and thoroughly combined.

Recommendations for use: Consume 15–20 minutes prior to exercise.

12. RELIEVES NAUSEA

Nausea is an unpleasant and uncomfortable sensation in the stomach that is often accompanied by the urge to vomit. As the body struggles to deal with the source of the issue (migraine, stress, etc.) physically, nausea can actually be a great indication that calls your attention to a need your body is desperately trying to fulfill. While the urge to combat the nausea with remedies like saltines and ginger ale may seem enticing, the answer may lie in a simple stub of ginger root.

For years, ancient cultures have remedied stomach ailments with the ginger root in a variety of tonics, tinctures, and chewables. With the addition of ginger to a carbonated beverage in the 1850s, the effectiveness of treating stomach upsets with ginger ale was surprising.

Unfortunately, today's ginger ales are only minimally effective because they rarely contain ginger, instead showering the stomach with harsh synthetics and sugars that exacerbate the issues. Fortunately, you only need to chew on a ½" × ½" slice of natural ginger for about 15–20 minutes to relieve your nausea. This releases the natural oils and phytochemicals in the ginger directly to the digestive system and into the bloodstream. Natural ginger provides a number of pH-balancing compounds that help to restore a natural balance of acids and enzymes to an upset stomach, while also providing analgesics that relieve pain. Also providing vitamins and minerals that can improve systems such as the cardiovascular, metabolic, and nervous systems that are directly related to the digestive system, the natural phytochemicals of ginger can improve the discomfort and nausea related to stomach upset by attacking the problem at its root while encouraging optimal performance of the systems directly related to it. Through the natural delivery of compounds that focus on returning the body to its healthy state, ginger can provide relief from nausea while also promoting the well-being of the brain and body!

THE HISTORY OF GINGER ALE

In 1851, the first ginger ale was created in Ireland, but it was a Canadian from Toronto named John McLaughlin who transformed the original dark, tasteless ale into the ginger ale we know and love today. Originally a pharmacist, McLaughlin got into the soda industry after purchasing a soda business and mixing fruit juices with carbonation. In 1890, he launched his "McLaughlin Belfast Style Ginger Ale," and went on to develop the paler "champagne of ginger ales" that is now known to nations across the world as "Canada Dry."

13. MINIMIZES MOTION SICKNESS

One out of every three people experiences some sort of motion sickness. Whether it results from a car ride, boat trip, or bus adventure, the dizziness, sweating, light-headedness, fainting, nausea, or vomiting that symptomize motion sickness can stop anyone from enjoying the most amazing of experiences . . . or even the simplest of commutes. While there are a number of commonly prescribed pills, potions, and pharmaceutical treatments, there can be a concern with the ingredients that may cause more harm than good. The chemicals, additives, and unhealthy ingredients commonly contained in the majority of average over-the-counter and pharmaceutical treatments can cause adverse reactions that lead to far worse experiences than the symptoms of motion sickness. Fortunately, when you opt for an all-natural treatment like ginger, you can alleviate your motion sickness while also benefitting your body and overall health.

The compounds and oils of ginger not only calm the stomach and soothe the body's systems, but also provide support to the nervous system and mental functioning, both of which are directly involved with the middle ear, which is the actual source of motion sickness. Using ginger to provide relief by promoting optimal health and physical functioning will surely outperform any promises an over-the-counter treatment can provide! With proven success documented in a study of eighty sailors prone to motion sickness, powdered ginger consumed 30–60 minutes prior to sailing resulted in a 40 percent reduction of motion sickness symptoms. But while the powdered version worked well, chewing fresh slices of the root may be the most successful use of ginger to combat motion sickness. Because of the effectiveness most find with chewing gum to prevent motion sickness, combining the action of chewing with the stimulating effects of spicy ginger is theorized to reduce the incidence of motion sickness exponentially.

14. CALMS FOOD POISONING

Surprisingly, one out of every six Americans suffers from some form of food poisoning every single year. There are more than 250 possible different causes to blame for the development of the dreaded condition, and the most common can be traced to eating expired or exposed food harboring bacteria that wreaks havoc on the digestive and immune system. While most cases of food poisoning are characterized by symptoms like nausea, vomiting, headaches, muscle aches, fatigue, confusion, and diarrhea, the more severe forms can be harmful enough to cause kidney failure, chronic arthritis, brain and nerve damage, or even death.

While serious cases should seek medical attention immediately, ginger can be used to treat the symptoms and relieve the underlying causes of minor cases of food poisoning. Not only can the cause of food poisoning be effectively "flushed out" and treated internally, but the body can be returned to a healthy state naturally with the use of ginger. By improving digestion and metabolism with its unique acid-combatting and pH-balancing enzymes and oils, restorative vitamins and minerals like vitamin C, calcium, and magnesium, and replenishing probiotic effects, ginger can actually assist the body in processing the bacteria that caused the food poisoning, helping to move the body into repair faster. In addition, ginger's electrolytes, and the additional phytochemicals that increase the body's absorption of those electrolytes, help the body begin the reparation process faster and more efficiently. And, with its immunity-boosting elements, ginger can also help relieve the symptoms of food poisoning and safeguard your weakened immune system from illnesses that could thrive in a body weakened by sickness.

SEEK MEDICAL ATTENTION

The American Association of Poison Control urges sufferers to report their cases of food poisoning to their hotline—1 (800) 222-1222—and to seek immediate medical attention if symptoms worsen or do not subside after 3–5 days.

15. RELIEVES HEARTBURN

Heartburn is described as the uncomfortable burning sensation that affects the esophagus, sometimes accompanied by an acidic taste in the mouth or even a small amount of acidic bile being expelled into the mouth. Sometimes, heartburn, which is actually a symptom, can be a result of a simple bacterial infection in the stomach or a common side effect of frequently prescribed medications such as aspirin, steroids, estrogen (birth control), or those intended to treat blood pressure, cholesterol, or thyroid conditions. Heartburn can also be as simple as an adverse physical reaction to the consumption of spicy food or caffeine, engaging in smoking or alcohol consumption, or experiencing excessive stress or indigestion. Beyond the adverse reactions' symptoms, heartburn can also be an indicator of more serious conditions like irritable bowel syndrome (IBS), ulcers, gallstones, or GERD.

Regardless of the condition that may precipitate the onset of heartburn, ginger can help reduce the severity of the experience while providing the body with a number of healing components that can not only improve the physical reaction, but actually encourage the repair of most underlying conditions. Ginger's balancing pH helps return the overly acidic state of your stomach contents to a normal level, helping alleviate the immediate cause and discomfort of heartburn. With the vitamins, minerals, oils, enzymes, and phytochemicals provided by ginger, the body can begin a repairing process that helps the digestive, circulatory, cardiovascular, and nervous systems, all of which are intertwined in the serious conditions that can produce heartburn as a symptom, and not merely a simple adverse reaction. Luckily, even if the cause of the heartburn is a simple upset or unbalance that has produced an isolated situation of heartburn, chewing a simple slice of ginger or sipping a spicy cup of ginger-infused green tea (see the "Reduces Bitter Flavors in Food and Drink" entry later in this chapter for a recipe) can provide on-the-spot relief in the most delicious possible way!

16. MINIMIZES MORNING SICKNESS

Pregnancy is one of the most delightful and anticipated parts of life. However, within the first few weeks of a pregnancy, another not-so-desirable feeling can quickly turn previously perfect mornings into ones plagued with nausea and vomiting that ebb and flow without warning. The largest contributor to the onset of morning sickness is the fluctuation of hormones flowing throughout the newly pregnant body. With these high levels of hormones come sensitivities to smells, constipation or diarrhea, fluctuations in mood and emotions, and a number of physiological reactions in the body and brain that can create a "perfect storm" of uneasy or uncomfortable situations that directly affect the digestive system.

Ginger has been one of the most commonly prescribed morning sickness relievers for centuries, and can actually help relieve the unpleasant symptoms associated with morning sickness while also promoting the health of almost every system related to the healthy development of a baby. Providing B vitamins and folate, ginger not only helps regulate the hormonal balance of the mother and promote the healthy growth of the fetus, but helps prevent the folate-deficient condition known as spina bifida in the fetus. Amino acids, oils, and phytochemicals also promote the absorption of the essential vitamins and minerals required by the mom and baby during pregnancy, reducing the risk of the deterioration of the mother's stores of minerals (like calcium) to supply the baby's needs. With the combination of a calming effect on morning sickness and the provision of necessary nutrients, phytochemicals, oils, and enzymes that support the healthy growth of both mom and baby, ginger is the perfect go-to for any mom-to-be hoping to make the best out of a pregnancy . . . and her baby's future.

CONSULT A PHYSICIAN?

Even with new warnings that claim expectant mothers should "consult a physician" before consuming ginger during pregnancy, there are no documented scientific cases of this all-natural herb causing unhealthy reactions in moms or fetuses.

17. NATURALLY INCREASES APPETITE

Surprisingly, a growing number of circumstances and conditions have increased the percentage of people searching for a product that can naturally stimulate their appetite without adverse side effects. Suffering most from the conditions requiring an increase in appetite are the elderly, who commonly experience lack of appetite due to medications, lack of interest in eating alone, chewing challenges that result from arthritis or dentures, or depression. The elderly aren't the only ones who find themselves prescribed with a more nutrient-dense diet, however; people of all ages who report traumatic situations, stress, depression, or nervousness can find themselves with a fading eagerness to follow dietary guidelines.

Not surprisingly, ginger's naturally spicy flavor can actually improve the experience of eating by stimulating one's senses. And, since ginger naturally stimulates the metabolism and the digestive system, the body will sometimes react to the introduction of ginger by craving foods that contain the nutrients it needs, like iron-rich spinach or fructose-full fruits. These depleted stores of vitamins and minerals are not only satisfied with the nutritious foods that are consumed, but ginger aids in increasing the absorption and metabolism of those nutrients, which helps the body store, utilize, and deliver the nutrients throughout the body. With the added benefit of mental stimulation through the delivery of B vitamins, ginger can help revive a natural interest in foods while also providing the energy needed to exercise; not only does this help stimulate and support all of the systems related to healthy eating, but the resulting calorie burn can also spike an interest in calorie-dense foods. Naturally and gradually, ginger can help anyone dealing with suppressed appetite to learn to love food again!

18. REDUCES BITTER FLAVORS IN FOOD AND DRINK

Adding a spicy food to a tea, tonic, or dish to reduce bitter flavors may sound simply crazy. But in the same way that salt can intensify sweet flavors or citrus can brighten sensational cream sauces, the uniquely spicy flavor of the ginger root can lend a calming twist to otherwise bitter dishes and drinks. One amazing way to experience this method is with green tea.

TO MAKE 1 POT OF GREEN TEA, USE:

Water (enough to fill 1 tea pot)
8 green tea bags
1–3" ginger root

Bring the water to a boil, then remove from the heat. Place the tea bags in the tea pot, and add the boiled water. Cover the pot while you peel the 1–3" piece of ginger and slice it into 1" pieces of ginger to provide for maximum surface area. After the ginger is prepared, remove the lid from the pot, add the ginger to the hot water and tea bags, and replace the lid. Allow the covered tea to cool on the stove for a minimum of 6–8 hours, which will allow the ginger to infuse throughout the tea.

Recommendations for use: Whether you prefer to drink the tea chilled or hot, the slight spiciness of the ginger should permeate throughout every sip, cutting the naturally bitter flavor of the green tea almost completely.

Because of the naturally occurring oils in ginger, the addition of this root should be as fresh as possible to ensure maximum flavor and benefits. Keeping in mind that the promotion of almost every body's proper functioning results from the addition of ginger to the diet, the simple and spicy addition that heightens flavor while minimizing bitterness should be greatly appreciated from not only a culinary standpoint, but in the pursuit of health as well.

REMOVE THE RESIDUE

When green tea is brewed, the health benefits can be extraordinary, but the natural flavors can sometimes be bland, bitter, and leave an unpleasant aftertaste. When boiling water for the green tea, be sure that no residue remains in the pan from previous dishes; even the slightest film or residue from pasta, sauces, or past tea preparations can leave a slight flavor that will alter the natural taste of the green tea.

19. IMPROVES THE SPICY FLAVORS OF FOOD

When you're preparing a meal that you hope will have complexity, deliciousness, and a "wow factor" to impress your guests, you need look no further than ginger to help. This ingredient not only helps brighten and embody the naturally spicy flavors of a dish, but ginger's ease of use and versatility only intensifies the desire to try the root in any number of ways! Why should you try using this delicious addition in one of your meals to add a little extra spice that also packs a ton of nutrition and health benefits as soon as possible? Well, ginger can add sweetness or spiciness, depending upon how it is prepared prior to use. The recipe here utilizes the ginger root's spicy flavor and can add flavor to any dish with which it's served.

TO MAKE ABOUT 2 CUPS OF SPICY PICKLED GINGER, USE:

8 ounces fresh ginger, peeled and sliced thin or shaved

2 tablespoons minced jalapeño, ribs and seeds removed

1 teaspoon fine sea salt

1 cup rice vinegar

¼ cup honey

1. In a small dish, combine ginger, jalapeño, and sea salt. Toss to coat.
2. Transfer ginger and jalapeño to an airtight jar with a tight-fitting lid.
3. In a small saucepan over medium heat, combine the rice vinegar and honey, bring to a boil stirring constantly, and remove from heat.
4. After vinegar-honey solution has cooled for 30–40 minutes, pour into the jar of ginger and jalapeño, top with lid, and shake to combine well.

Recommendations for use: Store in refrigerator for one week before consuming.

20. DETOXIFIES AND REJUVENATES THE LIVER

For those in search of a delicious detoxification, the Spicy Green Detox Smoothie is here! With the addition of ginger, this smoothie provides ample amounts of enzymes that not only encourage detoxification throughout the body, but detoxify and rejuvenate the liver for improved efficiency when detoxing! This smoothie also includes nutrient-dense greens and fruits that provide powerful vitamins and minerals, along with a host of naturally occurring phytochemicals that help rid the body of waste and toxins. Combined with these healthy ingredients, ginger ensures that this smoothie is a simple and easy way to encourage the detoxification process naturally.

TO MAKE 2 CUPS OF THE SPICY GREEN DETOX SMOOTHIE, USE:

1 cup spinach leaves

2 kale leaves

1" piece of ginger, peeled

1 Fuji apple, cored and peeled

1 cup organic apple juice (not from concentrate)

1 frozen banana, peeled

Combine all ingredients in a blender, then blend until all ingredients are emulsified and thoroughly combined.

Recommendations for use: Drink immediately, storing remaining smoothie in an airtight container in the refrigerator for up to 4 hours.

21. PACKS NUTRIENTS INTO SUPER-GREEN GINGER-PEAR SMOOTHIE

With smoothies acting as the perfect snack option at home or on the go, there's no easier way to consume a daily serving of fruits and vegetables! Supporting every one of the body's systems and functions through the plentiful provisions of nutrients and phytochemicals, this smoothie recipe combines the spiciness of ginger with the sweetness of pears, blended perfectly with antioxidant-rich spinach and kale for a double dose of greens that pack a punch of essential vitamins and minerals the body needs to achieve optimal health and maintain optimal functioning. The contributions to the taste or health benefits provided by the ginger are pretty impressive, considering the small amount included in the recipe. Packed into the 1" piece of ginger is a wide variety of powerful antioxidants, anti-inflammatory agents, stimulating vitamins, nourishing minerals, and a number of potent phytochemicals that support the health of the body's cells, tissues, organs, and systems. With all of the deliciousness packed into this smoothie, you might even forget how healthy it is!

TO MAKE 2 CUPS OF THE SUPER-GREEN GINGER-PEAR SMOOTHIE, USE:

1 cup spinach leaves
2 kale leaves
2 pears, cored
1" piece of ginger, peeled
2 cups organic apple juice (not from concentrate)

Combine all ingredients in a blender and blend until thoroughly combined.

Recommendations for use: Drink immediately, storing remaining smoothie in an airtight container in the refrigerator for up to 4 hours.

22. CLEANSES THE PALATE

With spicy and sweet notes that awaken the senses, ginger is a little-known palate cleanser that can effectively remove the residual tastes from foods or drinks, reviving the palate and allowing for the full effect of new flavors to be experienced. While some people are unaware of this magnificent aspect of ginger, ancient cultures have utilized the root for this specific purpose for thousands of years. In addition to the benefit to be gained from utilizing ginger in culinary situations where palate-cleansing allows for multiple tastings of various courses or dishes, ginger can also be used to remove undesirable tastes from the tongue and mouth that can result from any number of common situations such as poorly paired ingredients, undesirable flavor combinations, or an adverse physical reaction resulting in abnormal salivary or digestive responses.

Cleansing the palate is not only important in dining situations, but can be an effective method in preventing bad breath, minimizing digestive dysfunctions such as acid reflux with its pH-balancing capabilities, and reducing the incidence of bacterial and viral overgrowths that can contribute to the "bad taste" experience. All you need is a 1" slice of fresh ginger, and you can chew or suck on the antimicrobial and digestive system–soothing root, which will help deliver health-promoting properties directly where they're needed in order to combat undesirable tastes. While clearing the mouth of germs, bacteria, and undesirable flavors, ginger's sweet and spicy taste can also improve the production of saliva, helping to ensure the mouth remains clear and refreshed safely and naturally.

THE CLEANSING POWER OF GINGER

For centuries, Asian culture has utilized ginger for its cleansing benefits that protect against infiltration and spread of bacteria, virus, and microbes. While modern society has grown accustomed to having ginger served aside their favorite Asian cuisine, few realize that the original intention of this ginger accompaniment was to rid the mouth of foul-tasting organisms that could taint the taste of the cuisine. There's no question, cleansing the palate of bad taste while cleansing the body of toxins and harmful organisms never tasted so good.

Chapter 2

TOTAL WELLNESS

The systems within the body work synergistically, depending upon one another for support. Because this network is so well integrated, a dysfunction in any system can quickly result in a cascade of dysfunctions throughout the body. When these dysfunctions occur, the first signs are the physical symptoms that can include anything and everything from inflammation to fatigue, weight loss to weight gain, or serious conditions such as illnesses and disease. In an effort to live a full life that's free of dysfunction and disease, you only need to focus on providing your body with all that it needs, while protecting it from the risk factors that pose potential harm.

Fortunately, by supplying your body with ginger, you are able to benefit from a number of naturally occurring phytochemicals that not only promote health, but protect it. With the simple addition of a single serving of ginger, whether it be ¼ teaspoon of powdered or 1 tablespoon of dried, pickled, or fresh, the benefits to the entire body can be experienced, helping you to achieve optimal health naturally and with minimal effort (and great taste!). Through the abundant supply of unique oils, enzymes, and nutrients (some of which come only from the ginger root), every one of the body's systems benefit, leading the entire network to function optimally. Simply, naturally, safely, and effectively, ginger can help reverse, repair, restore, and protect your health . . . all while adding sweetness and spice to your life!

23. INCREASES ENERGY

Ginger is one of the few time-tested traditions that has remained a natural go-to when it comes to energy production. For centuries, the root has been boiled down and mixed into tonics and tinctures to be taken by the soldier on the battlefield and the everyday man or woman at home who needs an extra "oomph" in their step. Until recently, though, ginger was thought to be somewhat of an old wives' tale in terms of its capabilities in fighting fatigue, improving mental functioning, or increasing and sustaining energy levels. Now, however, it has been scientifically proven that ginger can not only increase energy levels, but can also support the body's systems as they obtain, convert, utilize, and sustain energy for use in every way imaginable.

When you add ginger to your diet, you unharness an unimaginable amount of naturally occurring polyphenols that seep into the digestive system, and are directed throughout the bloodstream to every cell, organ, and system. When this occurs, the different oils, enzymes, and nutrients in ginger begin a cascade of reactions that lead to improved metabolic functioning, increased cardiovascular functioning, and better communication within the nerve cells throughout the body, including the brain. With this increase in activity, the body and brain experience a heightened ability to convert food to energy and supply those stores to the areas in need, all while supporting the very systems that utilize that energy for fuel.

24. IMPROVES MEMORY

With every aspect of ginger's benefits being explored to a new degree by the way of modern medicine, a new light has shone on the advantages of adding ginger to a diet in reference to memory. In multiple studies performed on hundreds of male and female participants, ginger was given in doses ranging from 400–800 mg per day, and compared with a placebo. Astoundingly, participants who received the ginger extract, *Zingiber officinale*, outperformed the participants who were given a placebo when presented with memory tests. Increasing the surprise of the results, the participants who received the ginger extract actually *improved* their performance on memory testing throughout the trial, as opposed to the participants given the placebo, who received fluctuating, and less superior, performance grades on their testing. These impressive results were even more startling, as the participants had only been administered the ginger extract for a period of two months!

While the specific aspects of ginger that contribute to the improvement of memory storage and retrieval have not been thoroughly identified, there are enzymes and oils within ginger that are thought to have a direct effect on the functioning of the nerve cells and brain matter responsible for memory.

THE SCIENCE BEHIND GINGER'S ABILITY TO IMPROVE MEMORY

A 2010 study conducted by the Department of Neuroscience Program's faculty at Khon Kaen University in Thailand explored the science behind ginger's positive effects on memory and determined that the antioxidant activity of the oils within the ginger root safeguards the neurons of the brain (including those directly related to memory) from damage resulting from oxidative stress, illness, or physical damage. During this particular study, rats who had experienced cerebral ischemia (known to produce brain damage affecting cognitive functioning and memory) were administered ginger's oils in the form of an alcohol extract prior to and following the onset of the condition; these rats not only outperformed the control group in cognitive functioning, but also showed a "cognitive enhancing effect and neuroprotective activity."

25. SHARPENS MENTAL CLARITY

Have you ever experienced that "scattered" feeling, when you have so many things to focus on that you can't focus on anything? Surprisingly, it may not be just the countless items on your to-do list that are making you unable to see one task through to completion. Instead, the chemical reactions and responses occurring in your brain and throughout your body may be responsible for running interference. Hormone fluctuation, metabolic functioning, neuron communication, and circulatory system health are four of the most common factors that affect mental clarity. Knowing this, new and exciting research is showing conclusively that you can improve your mental functioning and clarity through easy, effortless care using none other than ginger.

Providing your body with the fuel required to function properly is one of the most essential keys to improving mental clarity. Without the adequate carbohydrates, proteins, and fats that the body and brain require to function, every system is adversely affected, especially the brain. Helping to rectify these situations, ginger provides your body with the essential nutrients, micronutrients, and amino acids that are required for proper brain and nerve system functioning. Further promoting the brain's optimal functioning, ginger's unique oils and phytochemicals improve circulation and regulate hormones and blood sugar levels, ensuring the brain and body maintain levels conducive to optimized mental functioning. With the added benefit of powerful antioxidants that have shown to protect against dangerous cell changes such as oxidation or degradation, ginger is even able to safeguard the brain and the body from serious conditions that can complicate mental processes, keeping your mind and body free and clear!

26. FIGHTS DEPRESSION

A staggering 350 million people world-wide will experience depression at some point in their lives, according to the World Health Organization. Attributed with the largest number of people requiring attention for a con-dition severe enough to be labeled a "disability," depression is a growing concern that affects almost every per-son, regardless of age, gender, or socio-economic status. With mood swings, bouts of depressive episodes that can only be described as severe sadness, loneliness, or despair, and suicidal thoughts, depression is not something that should be taken lightly, so be sure to educate yourself on the topic and don't hesitate to set up an appointment with a doctor before jumping to a self-diagnosis of the disorder.

While depression can be attributed to trauma, grief, injury, or life experiences, there are a number of studies that show that the chemical reactions in the brain—and the hormones released as a result—may directly affect the severity of a depressive episode, and be responsible for the "episode" extending into a "condition." In one study, scientists added ginger to the diets of participants who otherwise experienced multiple or long-lasting periods of depression in a three-month period of time. When compared to participants who were given a placebo, the participants with ginger reported fewer depressive episodes and more consistent days without symptoms characterizing the condition. Through these multiple trials, researchers have been able to conclude that ginger's effects on the brain's chemistry, the body's production of hormones, and the impact on the synergistic systems that promote energy and "happiness" are effective in treating depression.

27. ACTS AS A NATURAL AROMATHERAPY AID

Aromatherapy is the use of aromatic plant extracts for therapeutic purposes, including stress relief and the promotion of feelings of peace and contentedness. While it might seem somewhat silly to think that a simple smell could provide an experience that changes the mind, mood, or sense of self, ample research supports the effectiveness of using sensory activation in an effort to stimulate the senses with specific responses to specific smells. While some aromas promote energy, vigor, and stimulation, others can produce a contrary reaction like relaxation, calm, and even sustained sleep. Regardless of the mood you may be experiencing at any given moment, a simple whiff of the right aroma can transfix your senses, shifting your mood, your mind, and your body to the way you *want* to feel, instead.

With the unique spiciness that can only be provided by ginger, a simple scrape of the exterior of a ginger root unleashes an aroma that is as versatile as it is pungent. While other aromas fall into specific categories that either stimulate or subdue the senses, ginger is able to be used for either purpose!

Whether you choose to naturally awaken your body and mind with a tincture of ginger oil in the morning or by simply scraping or juicing the root, you harness your midday energy for enhanced focus and productivity with the delightful ginger-infused mist sprays included in the "Energizes Skin" and "Revitalizes Skin" entries in Chapter 3, or soothe yourself to sleep with the same delightful tincture's juiced drops at night, ginger can provide you with mood-boosting benefits that permeate your day and night, for an experience beyond compare!

28. IMPROVES CIRCULATION

Millions of people around the world experience poor circulation, which is characterized by tingling, numbness, chills, temperature fluctuations, or recurrent episodes of extremities "falling asleep." The circulatory system delivers oxygen and all of the nutrients to the body's cells, organs, and systems. When this system is stressed by situations like the reduced flow of blood to or from the heart; excessive sodium, sugars, or fats in the bloodstream; or a deficiency in a nutrient that is required for the optimal functioning of the cardiovascular system and all of its parts, poor circulation can result. And, while the sensations that result from poor circulation (which is actually a symptom of a larger problem) can be unpleasant or even painful, the cause of this symptom can be downright deadly. Obesity, diabetes, and serious heart conditions are just a few examples of conditions that can contribute to the development of poor circulation, while also worsening the body's ability to promote healthy circulation. This endless cycle can lead to worsened poor circulation, eventually resulting in blockages within the arteries and blood vessels, increased blood pressure, heart attacks, and strokes.

Luckily, ginger has beneficial oils and phytonutrients that can not only improve your circulation, but ensure that proper circulation is promoted in a number of ways. Through their abilities to cleanse the blood, boost metabolism, regulate cholesterol levels, and maintain proper blood sugar levels, ginger's components not only promote proper circulation, but help to correct the pre-existing conditions that hinder it. With its effects on hormone levels and brain functioning, ginger can also help poor circulation sufferers maintain healthy habits like regular exercise through its naturally occurring phytochemicals, which work to increase energy levels, stimulate senses, maximize metabolic functioning, and maintain proper cardiovascular and nervous system health, which can not only improve circulation, but help achieve and maintain an optimal health level!

29. HELPS RELIEVE HYPERTENSION

Hypertension is a well-known condition that refers to a consistent state of high blood pressure. There are two types of hypertension: primary and secondary. Primary hypertension is also known as "essential" and develops gradually over time, while secondary hypertension appears suddenly due to the onset of a condition such as kidney or thyroid problems, congenital defects, medications, or drug and alcohol abuse.

Normal blood pressure is considered to be a systolic rate (the top number of your blood pressure reading that evaluates the pressure within your arteries when your heart beats) of less than 120, while hypertensive refers to a blood pressure between 120 and 139, or higher.

While a number of medications can alleviate hypertension, many physicians recommend a change in diet that minimizes salt, sugar, and unhealthy fat, and maximizes consumption of whole fruits and vegetables, healthy fats, and whole grains. Fortunately, you can add ginger to your daily routine for astounding benefits that not only directly affect blood pressure, but improve the overall functioning of the body, ensuring maximum support for the cardiovascular system and blood pressure regulation.

The naturally occurring polyphenols, which are plant-based nutrients, chemicals, and compounds contained within ginger, have shown to lower overall blood pressure (which is why it is *never* recommended to consume ginger when taking medications prescribed for high blood pressure conditions). Through an effective reduction of LDL cholesterol (the "bad" cholesterol), ginger's compounds are able to help prevent the plaque buildup in the blood, blood vessels, and arteries thought to contribute to minimized blood flow and circulation. It also supports the body's metabolism and circulation of blood throughout the body, which not only assist the cardiovascular system's functioning, but also directly affect the rate and flow of blood pressure throughout the body.

GINGER'S USE WITH MEDICATIONS IS NOT RECOMMENDED WITHOUT APPROVAL

Because a daily dose of ginger can deliver benefits to the body that result in drastically changed blood sugar levels, hormone levels, and triglyceride and cholesterol levels, it is absolutely essential for any patient undergoing treatment for blood-related conditions to consult their physician before adding ginger to their daily routine.

30. IMPROVES THE FUNCTION OF THE CARDIOVASCULAR SYSTEM

Most people are unaware of the amazing functions, processes, and procedures for which the cardiovascular system is responsible. Consisting of the heart, blood vessels, and approximately 5 liters of blood, the cardiovascular system is responsible for transporting oxygen, nutrients, hormones, sources of cellular energy, and products of cellular waste to wherever they need to go throughout the body. With every minute that passes, the cardiovascular system is able to pump the body's 5 liters of blood through the heart to the body and back to the heart again!

The most effective way to support healthy functioning of the cardiovascular system is to focus on improving your lifestyle. Reducing stress; avoiding cigarettes, drugs, and alcohol; daily cardiovascular exercise and regular strength training; maintaining a clean diet free of excess salt, sugar, and unhealthy fats; and ensuring you receive quality sleep every night are all essential components of a healthy cardiovascular routine. However, you can also add ginger to your diet and promote the health of your heart through the maintenance of a healthy body and mind.

With essential vitamins like B-'s, C, and K, and minerals like iron, calcium, potassium, and magnesium that help with cell functioning and nerve functioning, ginger actually helps the cardiovascular system by supporting some of the major components that ensure the heart is able to function correctly and produce the blood flow throughout the body as needed. With additional compounds that help the heart and body maintain clean blood, assist in heart rate and circulation, and metabolize waste products efficiently, the strain on the cardiovascular system as a whole is reduced with the addition of ginger. The stress of fluctuated hormones can also contribute to strain on the cardiovascular system, which is why a source like ginger that promotes proper hormone levels, as well as "feel-good" hormones like serotonin and dopamine in the brain, is essential in maintaining cardiovascular health.

31. PROMOTES PROPER BLOOD CLOTTING

Blood clotting, also known as coagulation, is the body's natural process of preventing excessive bleeding when a blood vessel has been injured. Through the joint effort of platelets, specialized blood cells, and proteins in the plasma—the liquid component of the blood—clots are formed, preventing excessive blood flow that could lead to death. Ensuring the body's ability to properly produce blood clots in response to injury, and slowly degrade those clots once the healing process is complete, is extremely important. If a blood clot is formed in a vein and is not dissolved by the cardiovascular system, a condition known as deep vein thrombosis can occur. If the blood clot remains undissolved and releases within the vein, that clot can travel to the brain, heart, or lungs, and cause a deadly embolism.

With the unique compounds of ginger, the body can better maintain healthy blood flow, proper circulation, delivery of essential nutrients to the blood's cells, and a blood quality that is necessary for the process of clotting. Through the addition of ginger's vitamins, minerals, phytonutrients, enzymes, and oils, the body can specifically promote proper blood clotting, while also optimizing the healthy functioning of the systems directly related to the process like the cardiovascular and nervous systems, as well as metabolic functions like hormone production and blood sugar regulation. Add ginger's capability to maximize the body's absorption of essential nutrients of a healthy diet to the mix, and consider the fact that ginger helps increase energy, metabolism, and hormone production, which have all proven to improve fitness levels, and you can clearly see that ginger is an important ally in the promotion of proper blood clotting.

POOR BLOOD CLOTTING

Because people over the age of 50 are at highest risk for improper blood clotting, researchers have tried to determine if the body suffers from specific age-related conditions that can affect the body's ability to properly clot and degrade those clots. While age itself is not a factor, certain lifestyle habits such as diet and exercise, as well as prescription medications, have shown to increase the prevalence of poor blood clotting.

32. IMPROVES BONE STRENGTH

The skeletal system is one of the most important support systems in the body that help to maintain overall health. This system provides structural support that allows your body to move, protects your organs against injury, and ensures that the body has ample amounts of calcium and other essential minerals at its disposal. In order to achieve and maintain healthy bones, a healthy lifestyle is a must! To benefit your bones, you need to eat a diet that provides ample amounts of the nutrients like iron, calcium, magnesium, and potassium that are required by the bones and their supporting systems, combined with a fitness-focused routine, adequate sleep, and reduced stress. You should also avoid any of the lifestyle habits that wreak havoc on your body's systems and functions (like smoking and alcohol consumption) and you've got the perfect combination of bone-building health.

In addition to these lifestyle choices and to maximize the strength of your bones, simply add ginger to your everyday routine. With its provisions of vitamins and minerals that contribute to bone health; enzymes that help to improve the absorption of the bone-building and strengthening mineral (calcium) obtained through a sound diet; phytochemicals that assist in the manufacturing and repair of collagen, thus helping bones maintain the necessary elasticity to prevent breakage; and energy-promoting properties that help to keep the body in motion and ensure it stays in motion, your skeletal system will be working at 100 percent before you know it! Powdered, raw, juiced, or whole, ginger is one must-have dietary addition that will not only spice up your diet, but keep your bones strong, too!

33. PROMOTES PROPER NERVE FUNCTION

The nerves participate in every single thought, reaction, motion, and function that takes place throughout your body. When you react to the touch of a burning pot, your nerves send a message to your brain, process that message within the brain, and then send a message back to the body, creating the split-second reaction of removing your hand from the pot. In addition, whenever you take a breath, your heart beats, your digestive system moves food through your body, or you experience a fluctuation in your body's temperature, nerves are involved.

The four major classifications of nerves are:

1. *Cranial:* communicate between the brain and sense organs
2. *Central:* communicate between the brain and spinal cord
3. *Peripheral:* communicate between the spinal cord and limbs
4. *Autonomic:* communicate between the brain and spinal cord with the organs (such as the stomach, intestines, and blood vessels)

Nerve functioning is just one more area of health in which ginger can help. Multiple researchers around the world have studied a number of ginger's dietary components and their effects on nerve functioning, and have determined that the compounds most effective in safeguarding nerve health and promoting proper functioning are the B vitamins; calcium, iron, and magnesium; omega-3 fatty acids; and the amino acids. As you know, ginger not only provides these very elements, but also contains rich sources of unique oils, enzymes, and phytochemicals that directly promote the systems and functions in which nerves are so important. Through the maintenance of your body's systems, the promotion of nerve health, and the improvement of overall health that results from the addition of ginger to the daily diet, your body and mind can be functioning optimally for years to come!

34. PROVIDES NATURAL PAIN RELIEF

Throughout history, when dealing with pain relief, many cultures turned to natural pain treatment methods that focused on identifying the source of the pain and treating the cause, while also treating the discomfort that resulted. With herbs, diet, immobilization, and the administering of heat or cold to the area of concern, most painful conditions were treated successfully. Today, scientific advances have led more and more people to treatment options for pain that, while temporarily effective in "relieving" pain, may actually mask symptoms resulting from a condition requiring attention, and contribute to a multitude of side effects or the development of new conditions resulting from simply taking regularly prescribed pain medications. Over-the-counter medications, prescription medications, and natural pain techniques have been compared in many areas of pain relief treatments, and researchers have seen astounding results with natural healing methods that safely and effectively reduce pain, treat the condition-causing symptoms, and improve overall functioning of the body.

Ginger is one of the most widely used treatment methods for pain management. Researchers throughout cultures and across continents have discovered that the reduction of pain associated with injury, illness, and serious conditions can be minimized with the ingestion of ginger, as well as the application of ginger oils applied directly to the site of pain (see following recipe). With its wide array of phytochemicals, natural enzymes, and powerful unique oils, ginger is able to deliver immediate relief to a body in pain naturally and effectively with no side effects.

TO MAKE 1 APPLICATION, USE:

Freshly juiced ginger

OR A 1:1 RATIO OF:

Powdered ginger
Water

Recommendations for use: Soak a washcloth or cotton balls with freshly juiced ginger or a 1:1 ratio combination of powdered ginger and water. Place over the area where pain relief is needed for 30–60 minutes as often as necessary until pain subsides.

35. ALLEVIATES ARTHRITIS SYMPTOMS

Arthritis is one of the most widely diagnosed conditions in the world, and there are hundreds of medical conditions that fall under the classification of arthritis, with many sufferers being diagnosed with types like osteoarthritis, rheumatoid arthritis, or infectious arthritis. And, just as the diagnoses vary, this condition that strikes the musculoskeletal system at any area of the body can create a varying degree of pain that inhibits the life of the arthritic person to different degrees. While many arthritis sufferers turn to medications, prescriptions, and over-the-counter pain relievers, few find permanent relief from the pain. To worsen the scenario for these patients, many of the medications being prescribed as treatments can cause serious side effects or contribute to the adverse effects on systems, functions, and overall health.

One physician and researcher by the name of Dr. Srivastava of Odense University in Denmark conducted a pain management study to compare the effectiveness of non-steroidal anti-inflammatory drugs (NSAID pain relievers) to the effectiveness of ginger consumption when treating the arthritis pain suffered by patients. In this astounding study, he not only determined that the patients given ginger showed a "significant improvement in pain, swelling, and morning stiffness," but went on to identify why ginger was superior as an arthritis pain reliever. His study showed that not only do ginger's natural phytochemicals and unique oils block the formation of inflammatory compounds (prostaglandins) that create inflammation, they also produce an antioxidant effect that breaks down existing inflammation, helping the body to heal *and* protect against further inflammation and arthritis pain. With published research showing how this inexpensive, readily available, easy to prepare and consume spice can naturally reduce arthritis pain without the risk of dangers to any aspect of health, arthritis sufferers have been saved by the ginger root!

36. MINIMIZES JOINT PAIN

Joints are the parts of your body that connect one bone to the next. Throughout the human body, there are an astounding 360 joints! From the inner ear to the fingers and toes, these joints allow the body to function, participating in a network of movable and immovable systems that interact and coordinate the actions performed every moment of the day. The most common causes of joint pain are injury and the resulting inflammation. When injury or agitation occurs within one of the joints that is used regularly, the resulting inflammation can cause pain and discomfort that is easily aggravated by simple everyday movements. Luckily, though, the use of ginger can help to provide relief from joint pain as well as help with the healing process.

Ginger contains gingerol and shogaol, oils that do double-duty as enzymes that directly promote the repair and prevention of joint inflammation and pain. These starring phytochemicals not only help target the cause and site of inflammation, but can also improve the uncomfortable swelling that so often accompanies it. Additional phytochemicals contained within ginger promote proper circulation, which is essential in improving the delivery of nutrients to the site of joints in need, and carry away any infectious or inflammatory irritants that can contribute to the painful experience. While consuming a diet focused on whole foods, avoiding sodium or sugar, maintaining a healthy weight, engaging in regular exercise (because "a body in motion stays in motion"!), and avoiding injury, anyone who enjoys ginger on a regular basis can ensure that their joints remain pain-free!

37. MINIMIZES MUSCLE ACHES

A dull, lingering ache in the muscles that limits movement, or contributes to pain when movement occurs, is the characterization of the uncomfortable situation known as "muscle aches." While many people associate muscle aches with an overly strenuous workout, there are a number of situations that can contribute to the development of the experience, including injury, excessive strain, or systemic issues such as inflammatory diseases. While muscle pain is normally isolated to one specific area, an illness or viral infection such as the flu can also cause pain to be felt in multiple areas.

While the seriousness of muscle aches can be cause for concern, the majority of these conditions can be treated simply, easily, and naturally right at home with the all-mighty ginger! Simply mix up a ginger topical treatment.

TO MAKE 1 APPLICATION OF GINGER TOPICAL TREATMENT, USE:

¼ cup juiced ginger
¼ cup apple cider vinegar

Recommendations for use: Soak a compress with the mixture and apply it directly to the site of the muscle ache for 30 minutes at a time until ache subsides. Not only will this help to relieve the inflammation resulting from the irritation, but it will also encourage improved circulation, help remove the cause of the muscle ache (such as lactic acid buildup), and restore nutrients needed for repair. Helping to regulate the hormones and pain receptors that reduce the experience of pain, ginger also minimizes the painful aching of muscle aches effectively and naturally!

SEEK MEDICAL ATTENTION

The National Institute of Health (NIH) recommends using ice on the site of the muscle ache for 1–3 days following the onset of the pain, followed by heat applications for any pain that persists beyond three days. It is highly recommended that you see a physician if a muscle ache persists beyond three to five days. The NIH also recommends seeing a physician if the cause of the ache is unknown, or the ache is accompanied by a rash, redness, or swelling. Seek medical attention immediately if there is any stiffness of the neck or fluid retention in a specific area, or the inability to move the affected area becomes severe.

38. REDUCES THE INCIDENCE OF MIGRAINES

Thought to be caused by vascular constriction in the brain, which limits blood flow through the veins of the brain and body, migraines are extreme headaches characterized by sharp, pounding pains normally localized in one area of the head. For some people, migraines are prefaced by vision disruptions that may include seeing "auras" of light, spots, or bright orbs in the vision field, or experiencing overall blurred vision. Distorted vision can be further complicated with a sudden onset of fatigue, or physical symptoms like numbness or tingling in any area of the body. Migraine sufferers who regularly experience these intense headaches may require medication in order to prevent or negate the debilitating headaches, but take a chance with the development of dangerous side effects or dependence. In order to naturally cure migraines without medical interference, researchers have developed a theory that includes prevention and treatment. The main ingredient of this natural migraine treatment method is none other than ginger!

With its naturally occurring vitamins and minerals, paired with its ability to improve the body's ability to absorb and utilize those nutrients more effectively, ginger is able to improve the migraine condition by ensuring that adequate nutrients are delivered to the systems of the body and brain that may directly affect the conditions that produce migraine headaches. The improved circulation, corrected hormone imbalances (such as serotonin), and regulation of the body's metabolic functioning that result from ginger's provisions of phytochemicals, enzymes, and oils all improve the body's functioning and reduce the stress on the vascular areas thought to contribute to migraine development. With the added benefit of its histamine-fighting properties, ginger is also able to prevent the allergic reactions to food and environmental conditions that have also been theorized to contribute to migraine development. Through the addition of ginger to the daily diet, whether it be in a drink, smoothie, meal, or tincture, the benefits of ginger can be used to minimize migraines naturally and effectively!

39. RELIEVES TENSION HEADACHES

Characterized as a tightness in the head that is best described as a feeling of a tight band being constricted around the head, tension headaches, which affect an estimated 3 million people every year, can be a result of a number of physical factors. These factors include fatigue, stress, hormone fluctuation, dehydration, hypoglycemia, or excessive muscle tension throughout the neck, back, or body. While most people who experience tension headaches do so infrequently, some experience chronic tension headaches more than fifteen days of the month. Interestingly, women are more than twice as likely as men to experience chronic tension headaches.

Because tension of the muscles in the neck, back, legs, and arms can contribute to tension headaches and migraines, stretching and regular exercise can help alleviate tension and prevent or relieve tension headaches. Consuming a clean diet focused on whole foods free of sugar, sodium, milk, and gluten, and ensuring adequate sleep are also preventative measures for tension headaches, and one of the most effective additions to a daily routine for headache prevention is the consumption of ginger. With its ability to contradict histamine production, ginger can block allergy symptoms that may contribute to the development of a tension headache. The most notable benefit of ginger in fighting tension headaches, though, is its ability to improve circulation, regulate hormone production, and improve metabolic functioning. Through these systemic improvements, the fluctuations in hormones (thought to be the reason behind females reporting more tension headaches than males), regulation of blood sugar, and ensuring the proper circulation needed for oxygen delivery to the brain can be normalized. Ginger can improve the brain and body's reactions to the physical and environmental stressors that contribute to tension headaches. With the added benefit of improved serotonin production and increased energy, the stimulation provided by ginger's spiciness can support a more active lifestyle that can help to minimize the incidence of headache experiences.

40. PROMOTES HEALTHY SINUS FUNCTIONING

The sinuses are an essential part of the body's immune system, respiratory system, and structure of the face, and they provide the body with one of the first lines of defense against illness. They lie behind the forehead and cheeks, forming tunnels that bring air in through the nostrils to be delivered to the lungs. These tunnels are lined with a membrane and cilia that are designed to collect allergens, dirt, bacteria, and viruses from the air before they can wreak havoc on the body's systems. When the sinuses are functioning normally, the collected allergens are able to be disposed of naturally through the expelling of clear mucus, either by blowing the nose or being swallowed and dispelled naturally. When the sinuses dysfunction, however, the allergens collect in the sinus pockets and begin to breed bacterial or viral infections that quickly produce the well-known symptoms of sinus pressure, green mucus, fatigue, fever, and even body aches. Luckily for sinus dysfunction sufferers, there is growing evidence supporting an all-natural effective prevention and treatment method that can alleviate sinus problems for good.

Ginger's spiciness is able to stimulate the body's production of mucus, helping to clear the sinuses of infectious invaders and dispel them naturally through loosened mucus that may have previously been built up or blocked. With its antibacterial and antiviral properties, ginger's natural oils help to promote the body's immune system functioning, improving the body's defenses against possible infection. Stimulating the circulatory system and metabolism, the addition of ginger can also reduce the chances of developing physical symptoms such as fatigue, headaches, or muscle aches. Last, but not least, the antioxidants, anti-inflammatory agents, and antiseptic properties provided by ginger, as well as its ability to promote the body's absorption and use of those nutrients, have shown to directly support the body's immune and respiratory systems, which will help prevent the incidence of sinus infections in the future.

41. ALLEVIATES ALLERGY SYMPTOMS

According to the American College of Allergy, Asthma, and Immunology (ACAAI), a shocking 50 million people in the United States alone suffer from allergies. While most people think of itchy eyes and a runny nose when asked about allergies, it can be surprising to learn that these are the mildest of allergy symptoms. Running along a scale that ranges from mild to moderate to severe, allergy symptoms can be as simple as red and irritated eyes to muscle pains, vomiting, and even death.

A surprising prevention for allergies and their symptoms can be found in none other than the ginger root. With phytochemicals that have shown to play an extraordinarily effective role in reducing inflammation, ginger can be used to minimize the effects of allergens on the respiratory system, skin, and throughout the digestive system, helping alleviate the inflammation caused by almost all categories of allergies. With mucous membranes being adversely affected by almost all allergens, resulting in sneezing and coughing, it's no surprise that the spiciness of ginger can alleviate allergy symptoms through its ability to increase mucus production while also thinning the mucus; this allows the sinuses and lungs to more easily remove allergens from the body. Last, but not least, ginger has a direct effect on the production of histamine, helping the body to "calm" its reactions on a hormonal level before symptoms can even occur!

42. REDUCES ASTHMA SYMPTOMS

According to the National Heart, Lung, and Blood Institute (NHLBI), asthma is a long-term disease that involves inflammation and tightening of the airways in response to triggers in the environment that can range from dust to smoke, pet dander to pollen. With a growing field focused on the prevention and treatment of asthma, the surprisingly little that is known about the cause or cure for asthma and its symptoms can be frustrating. What researchers have determined is that there may be a genetic predisposition for the disease, and that there are a number of preventative measures that can be taken to reduce the incidence of asthma attacks. While medications are available and readily prescribed for the treatment of asthma, many have undesirable side effects, and their effectiveness in treating or resolving the disease is questionable.

One natural method of treatment for asthma that is growing in popularity among natural healing practitioners is ginger. With an ability to improve the cardiovascular, respiratory, and immune systems, ginger is able to improve the body's ability to cleanse the blood of pathogens, lung functioning, and the body's ability to fight infection.

All of these systemic improvements can help an asthma sufferer prevent the body's asthmatic symptoms in response to triggers such as allergens, smoke, environmental factors, and even certain foods. One theory also promotes ginger as an effective asthma symptom reliever that can help clear the respiratory tracts of allergens that could lead to an attack, through a thinning of the mucus in the sinuses and lungs that results from ginger's spiciness. With its natural anti-inflammatory oils, ginger's most effective attribute for preventing asthma symptoms is the ability to minimize the physical response of swelling, irritation, and inflammation of the airways, the specific physical symptoms directly responsible for the airway constriction characterized by asthma.

43. ALLEVIATES RESPIRATORY TRACT INFECTIONS

Respiratory tract infections, also known as RTIs, refer to bacterial and viral infections of the sinuses, throat, airways, nose, nasal passages, or lungs. The respiratory tract is divided into the upper and lower sections, and each has its own causes and symptoms when an infection occurs.

The upper respiratory tract consists of the nose, sinuses, and throat, and its most common infections include the common cold, tonsillitis, sinusitis, laryngitis, and the flu. When these conditions occur, the symptoms can include coughing, sneezing, stuffy or runny nose, sore throat, or headaches. The lower respiratory tract consists of the airways and lungs, and the most common infections are bronchitis, pneumonia, bronchiolitis, tuberculosis, and the flu. The most common symptoms experienced with lower respiratory tract infections include coughing, excessive phlegm and mucus production, chest congestion, an increased breathing rate, wheezing, and difficulty breathing. The differences between the upper and lower respiratory tract infections can be significant, but both can be improved with the simple addition of ginger.

With its powerful antibacterial and antiviral benefits, ginger is able to alleviate respiratory tract infections of all kinds, directly within the respiratory tract as well as through its promotion of a healthy immune system. Ginger helps minimize inflammation through its healthy provision of the unique oils gingerol and shogaol, which begin to alleviate respiratory infection symptoms at the site of the issue, wherever the infection is localized. And, with its ability to promote the healthy functioning of every system and function involved with the respiratory system, ginger can further alleviate associated symptoms. It is able to relieve headaches and muscle aches by improving circulation, relieve chest congestion and sinus pressure through anti-inflammatory and increased mucus production, and relieve pain associated with respiratory tract infections and their symptoms. By treating symptoms and speeding up your recovery time, ginger really is the one-stop shop for alleviating respiratory tract infections!

44. ACTS AS AN EXPECTORANT FOR CHEST CONGESTION

Chest congestion is one of the most common physical reactions to an infection or irritation affecting the respiratory system, and can be one of the most challenging to experience. Many people experience an upper respiratory tract infection initially, which is then followed with excessive chest congestion, even if no other lower respiratory tract infection symptoms exist. This excessive mucus production associated with chest congestion can lead to further physical symptoms including tightness, pressure in the lungs and chest, difficulty breathing, or wheezing. While the condition can be uncomfortable, the dangers of prolonged congestion can be severe; serious conditions such as bronchitis and pneumonia can develop from excessive, prolonged, untreated chest congestion, and the damage to the body and brain resulting from reduced oxygen flow to the lungs can manifest in a number of debilitating ways.

Fortunately, ginger is one of the most effective natural healing agents for chest congestion. Whether the congestion is in the early stages, accompanies another condition or illness, or has persisted long past the healing of that underlying condition or illness, ginger is able to deliver unique healing components that can help to dry up the congestion, expel the excess mucus, and relieve the organs and systems affected by the congestion. With unique antimicrobial, antiviral, and antibacterial properties provided by ginger's natural oils, enzymes, vitamins, minerals, antioxidants, and anti-inflammatory agents, ginger attacks the underlying issue or cause of the chest congestion, helping to improve the body's healing and inhibit the production of mucus. Providing anti-inflammatory properties, ginger can also improve the lungs' ability to process and expel mucus-causing agents that enter the respiratory system. And, it can even work to prevent the inflammation that contributes to and results from mucus production, putting a stop to a seemingly endless cycle that produces and continues congestion.

45. SOOTHES SORE THROATS

When dealing with health assailants like bacterial and viral infections, seasonal allergies, dry air, postnasal drip, or countless environmental factors such as smoke, dust, etc., a sore throat can be one of the body's first reactions. When dealing with a sore throat, it can be tempting to visit the nearest drugstore for a quick fix like any one of the wide variety of pills, potions, and sprays that promise to deliver relief. The catch with these over-the-counter treatments is that the ingredients can be questionable, the side effects can be worse than the original condition of a simple sore throat, and they seldom provide relief from the actual cause of the sore throat.

When you take ginger to treat your sore throat, you know what you're taking! Ginger is able to be consumed fresh, powdered, pickled, or stewed, and provides effective sore throat relief in any of those forms, and its anti-inflammatory compounds combine with its analgesic properties to reduce irritation and provide pain relief. In addition, powerful antimicrobial, antibacterial, and antiviral properties are not only delivered directly to the site of a sore throat after consuming ginger, but are distributed throughout the entire body via the digestive system, helping to relieve the throat and the entire body of the microbe or microbes responsible for the sore throat. Ginger's delivery of antioxidants through its many vitamins and minerals further supports the functioning of the immune system and promotes the prevention of the illnesses that can contribute to a sore throat, or provides relief and faster healing times when situations other than illness are responsible for the onset of the sore throat.

46. BOOSTS IMMUNE-SYSTEM FUNCTIONING

The immune system is your body's first line of defense against illness, and also multitasks as a support system to all of the body's organs and functions. Without an effective immune system, the body and all of its parts and procedures are vulnerable to potentially devastating conditions ranging from the common cold to serious cancers.

Ginger has begun to receive well-deserved attention in terms of its ability to promote healthy immunity. Providing antioxidants in the form of oils like gingerol and shogaol, in addition to its provisions of antioxidants, vitamins, and minerals, ginger is able to promote healthy cell growth and attack unhealthy cells. By providing the body's systems with adequate nutrition and superior protection, ginger helps the immune system protect against illness, the cardiovascular system focus on the organs and functions related to the blood and heart, and the nervous system focus on mental processes and cognitive functioning. These are just a few examples, but they illustrate how ginger's natural phytochemicals allow the body to function as designed, rather than expend energy on unnecessary illness or disease prevention.

In addition to antioxidants, ginger is a great source of vitamin C and zinc, which are both required for the proper functioning of the immune system's white blood cells, and with adequate numbers of blood cells and the improved performance of those blood cells resulting from sufficient nutrient delivery, the immune system is able to maintain proper functioning and effectively protect the body from illness, infection, or the development of disease. Added to these benefits is the fact that ginger has the capability of preventing and reversing inflammation, and provides the body with powerful antimicrobial properties to fight germs on contact. It's so easy to see how ginger can be an amazing addition to any life in need of immune system support!

HEALTHY CHOICES EQUAL HEALTHY LIVING

In addition to ginger, healthy lifestyle choices such as consuming a clean diet of nutrient-dense foods and avoiding sugars, sodium, and unhealthy fats; engaging in regular exercise; getting adequate sleep; keeping stress levels to a minimum; and refraining from alcohol and drug abuse and smoking all contribute to the development and maintenance of a strong immune system.

47. PREVENTS BACTERIAL INFECTIONS

Bacteria has existed on this planet for an estimated 3.5 billion years. Able to withstand extreme conditions like cold and heat, as well as radioactive environments, it's no wonder that the human body can play the perfect host. While most people hear "bacteria" and immediately think of infections, conditions, and diseases, only 1 percent of all bacteria are actually harmful. Actually, bacteria is required by the body in order to digest food, absorb nutrients, and even safeguard the body's organs and systems from the invasion and growth of disease-causing cells.

The smartest approach to bacteria is one in which the growth of good bacteria is promoted while the growth of bad bacteria is prevented. This may seem difficult, but the approach is actually quite simple when natural elements such as ginger are introduced to the body. While supporting healthy bacteria's growth and functioning with its enzymes and oils, but combatting the development of harmful bacteria naturally, ginger is able to safeguard the healthy aspects of the body's systems that depend on healthy bacteria (such as digestive flora) while negating those that could cause harm. With natural oils that actually seek and destroy harmful microbes and bacteria, ginger's ability to fight bad bacteria begins almost immediately upon entering the digestive system and bloodstream. One of the most amazing aspects of ginger can be seen when it is introduced to the body after a harmful bacterial infection has taken hold. This root is able to reduce fever through body temperature regulation, improve circulation and metabolism for the quick flushing of the invasive bacteria, and provide natural pain relievers that minimize aches and pains associated with infections. Ginger really is an all-in-one prevention and treatment that really works!

48. PREVENTS VIRAL INFECTIONS

Few people acknowledge, or are even aware, that viruses—like the ones that cause the dreaded flu—are everywhere, can be contracted quite easily, and are extremely difficult to eradicate once they have taken hold of a cell. The most intriguing aspect of viruses is that they are antibiotic-resistant, which means that those same medications and prescriptions that effectively treated another bacterial infection won't be able to treat a virus. And while vaccines have shown promise, there are questionable aspects about their side effects and effectiveness. Without question, the best defenses against viruses are to ensure that your immunity is optimal; be aware of the common symptoms of viral infections; start treatment as early as possible after infection; and to treat yourself naturally if and when a viral infection affects you. Luckily, ginger is able to save the day (and your body!) from viral infections and symptoms that can wreak havoc. Natural antiviral compounds are contained in every drop, sliver, and slice of the ginger root, and these compounds not only effectively attack the virus, but provide the body with antimicrobial and antibacterial support to help prevent further illnesses that could attack a compromised immune system. Helping to support the production of hormones, improve the digestive system's functioning, and regulate circulatory system functioning, ginger's compounds also minimize the severity of commonly associated symptoms such as fever and chills, nausea or vomiting, fatigue, and aches and pains.

49. COMBATS OVARIAN CANCER

Regarded as one of the deadliest forms of cancer, ovarian cancer is ranked as the fifth leading cause of cancer death among women. The American Cancer Society estimates that a woman's risk of developing ovarian cancer in her lifetime is 1 in 75, and a woman's risk of dying from ovarian cancer is 1 in 100. While the statistics seem to be favorable, the possibility of developing this deadly form of cancer is very real and warrants action that ensures the prevention or early diagnosis of this cancer, along with swift treatment. Regular health screenings and open communication with one's gynecologist can ensure that adequate preventative measures are in place, but major questions surround the steps necessary to ensure recovery if ovarian cancer has developed. With harsh cancer treatments providing questionable results, more physicians and patients are turning to natural treatment methods, and it's no surprise that ginger has taken the spotlight as one of the most promising natural treatment methods of the future.

In a 2006 University of Michigan study that explored the effectiveness of natural cancer treatment methods, ginger was researched as one of the experimental chemotherapy alternatives. Ginger, through its provisions of antioxidants, nutrients, and phytochemicals, was found to not only inhibit cancer cell growth throughout the female reproductive system, especially the ovaries, but was also determined to effectively support the body's functioning that would otherwise be compromised by the presence of cancerous cells and a weakened immune system. With researchers concluding that "ginger inhibits growth and modulates secretion of the angiogenic factors (the body's natural process of producing new blood vessels from existing vascular structures can be infiltrated with oxidative distress or cancerous growth, allowing for the illness or disease to spread rapidly) in ovarian cancer cells," growing attention is now being put into researching the effectiveness of using ginger as a cancer prevention or treatment in the future.

50. COMBATS RECTAL CANCER

Rectal cancer is the growth and spread of cancerous cells in the lower part of the colon that connects the large intestine to the anus. The rectum's primary function is to store formed stools in preparation for evacuation, making this area susceptible to a large number of toxins and waste that can collect and contribute to the cancerous growth within the surrounding walls of the rectum.

Within each of these layers, polyps (overgrowth of cells that protrude into the digestive tract and have a high probability of becoming cancerous or contributing to serious disease) can develop, collecting bits of waste that can produce inflammation and infection. Rectal cancer strikes 40,000 people every year in America, and 1.4 million people worldwide, making it the third most common type of cancer in the world, but few people are aware that this type of cancer is one of the most easily preventable forms—if the necessary precautions are put in place.

Through its unique blend of anti-inflammatory and anticarcinogenic properties, ginger is not only able to protect the rectum against dangerous changes such as inflammation, but it can also fight cancerous cell development before it starts. A recent study has identified one of ginger's oils, shogaol, as one that "induces cell death in colon and rectal carcinoma (cancer) cells." Though more research is being conducted in order to determine how to best use ginger's specialized oils for cancer prevention and treatment, the proven effectiveness of ginger in treating inflammation, evacuating toxins from the body, improving healthy cell growth, and attacking unhealthy or cancerous cells has shown promise as a possible natural treatment. Add to these benefits the fact that ginger is able to add healthy, cleansing fiber in the diet, and this root seems like an all-in-one resource for rectal cancer prevention.

SAFEGUARD THE RECTUM

The rectum's walls are made up of three layers:

- *Mucosa*: the innermost layer, composed of glands that secrete lubricating mucus that facilitates the movement of stools as they exit the body.
- *Muscularis Propria*: the middle layer, composed of muscles that contract in order to facilitate the forming of stools as well as their exit from the body.

- *Mesorectum*: the fatty tissue layer that surrounds the rectum and contains nerve cells that sense the presence of a prepared stool, and trigger the urge to release the stool.

With the buildup of waste's bacteria and harmful microbes settling in this system's multiple creases and crevices, it's easy to see how infections can fester and spread. With fiber-rich, antioxidant-packed ingredients like ginger added to the daily diet, the rectum can be safeguarded against illness and disease naturally and efficiently.

51. COMBATS COLON CANCER

Colon cancer is sometimes incorrectly grouped with rectal cancer, but these cancers affect completely different parts of the digestive system. The easiest way to clarify the difference between these two important parts of the digestive system is to simply state their responsibilities in the digestive process: the colon is where nutrients and water are absorbed from the food consumed, before the food is passed into the rectum, where it is formed into a stool to exit the body as waste. Because these areas are both involved in waste production, it's easy to understand how particles of waste can get left behind and create uncomfortable conditions like inflammation that can lead to dangerous illnesses and diseases.

By eating a diet rich in fiberful foods like greens, cruciferous vegetables, and fruits, the digestive system is thoroughly cleaned by a "goo" that is created when digestive enzymes meet with fiber. This goo fills the colon as it escorts foodstuff and waste throughout the process, ensuring that all bits and pieces are trapped and exit with the waste. However, detoxes, cleanses, and flushes are becoming more widely used methods for ensuring the colon stays free of debris and disease, and while these methods can be effective, some may be dangerous to the colon, leading to spasms, uncontrollable bowel movements, or dehydration, and may even lead to side effects or new conditions in other areas of the body. Fortunately, ginger not only provides the much-needed fiber that colons require for superior health, but the unique oils gingerol and shogaol help to fend off infections with their antioxidant capabilities *and* prevent unhealthy cancerous changes in the cells that line the colon's walls. With specialized phytochemicals that induce the death of colon cancer cells, prevent inflammation, and fight infection, the addition of ginger is a must for anyone experiencing colon troubles or who is at risk for colon cancer.

52. COMBATS SKIN CANCER

Skin cancer is a growing concern throughout the United States, and for good reason: In the past thirty years, the number of skin cancer diagnoses exceeded the number of all cancer diagnoses *combined*. According to the Skin Cancer Foundation, 5 million Americans are treated every year for skin cancer, with 2.8 million diagnosed with basal cell carcinoma (the leading form of skin cancer) and 700,000 diagnosed with squamous cell carcinoma. In fact, the diagnosis of squamous cell carcinoma has increased a staggering 200 percent in just three decades. These statistics show how prominent this condition is, but the statistic estimating that one person dies every 57 minutes from melanoma conveys how deadly the condition can be.

Without question, precautionary measures, early detection, and swift treatment can minimize the risk of developing dangerous skin cancer, but the addition of ginger has also shown to provide life-saving benefits for those who are in danger of developing the cancer or have already been diagnosed. Through the radio-protective properties that safeguard the cells against UVA and UVB rays, provided by the ginger's natural phytochemicals, the skin is protected from the carcinogenic effects of all of the ultraviolet rays. In addition, ginger's unique compound shogaol has been proven as an effective prevention/treatment option when introduced to the site of cancerous cells, either ingested or applied topically, since it's able to induce cell death specifically in carcinoma cells. When you combine this benefit with the antioxidant properties that naturally occur within ginger's oils, and also in its provisions of vitamins A, C, and E, the cancerous changes that occur within the cells in the development of cancer can be stopped, prevented, or even reversed.

STAY SAFE FROM SKIN CANCER

Heed the advice of the Skin Cancer Foundation and protect yourself from skin cancer by keeping your sun exposure minimal, wearing protective garments (especially during activities of prolonged sun exposure), and applying sunscreen and sunblock every day.

53. MINIMIZES TUMOR DEVELOPMENT

With each passing year, tumor diagnoses have been on the rise. Most people who have tumors are unaware of their presence until the growth undermines one of the body's organs or systems to the point where symptoms begin to arise. One important distinction between various types of tumors is whether they are benign or malignant. Benign tumors are not cancerous and, while they may grow in size, do not spread to surrounding cells or tissues. Malignant tumors are not only cancerous, but can invade and destroy healthy surrounding cells and tissues. Both tumor types can adversely affect the human body, but malignant tumors are far more concerning than the ones that are benign.

Ginger has been tested on tumors to determine whether its polyphenols (plant-based chemicals) can impact the cancerous and noncancerous growths. Not surprisingly, ginger has shown to halt the growth of malignant and benign tumors and, in some cases, has also caused cancerous cells in malignant tumors to die. In a 2010 study performed by the Department of Biotechnology and the BC Guha Centre for Genetic Engineering and Biotechnology at the University of Calcutta, ginger's sesquiterpene compound, zerumbone, was shown to "significantly raise the percentage of phagocytes, improving immune system functioning and reducing tumor growth." Further investigation allowed researchers to observe that ginger's compounds killed cancer by attacking the cancer cells specifically, and "reprogramming" the cancerous cells to destroy themselves; all of this cancerous cell death occurred alongside the preservation of healthy cells not affected by the cancer. Through its ability to kill cancerous cells and maintain healthy cell growth, ginger is growing in popularity as a possible tumor treatment in the very near future.

DECIPHERING CANCER ORIGINS AND SEVERITY

Tumors can develop in any tissue throughout the body; the tissue of origin gives the tumor its name. The most common tissues and the areas most affected or vulnerable to tumors are as follows:

- Connective: fat, cartilage, and bone
- Endothelium and mesothelium: blood vessels, lymph vessels, and mesothelium
- Blood and lymphoid cells: hematopoietic cells and lymphoid tissue
- Muscle: smooth or striated muscle
- Epithelial tissues: squamous, liver or kidney, placenta, or teste tissues

- Neural: glial or nerve cells, meninges, or nerve sheath

The profound capabilities of ginger's many potent compounds in the successful prevention and treatment of tumor growth, added to the multiple benefits to the brain and body's optimal functioning when ginger is consumed on a regular basis, leave no wonder as to why this age-old treatment is growing in popularity not only among consumers, but medical professionals as well.

54. MINIMIZES THE SIDE EFFECTS OF CHEMOTHERAPY

Deciding to undergo chemotherapy is a very difficult decision for cancer sufferers to make. On one hand, a cancer has to be killed in order for the patient to survive. On the other hand, chemotherapy is not always effective and has been shown to produce a number of life-altering side effects, including nausea, vomiting, colds and flus (due to the weakened immune system's ability to fight common microbes), excessive gas, fatigue, and intense joint pain. Fortunately, ginger has shown to drastically improve a number of the side effects, all while improving the functioning of the systems that support the healing from cancers.

As soon as ginger is consumed in the suggested amount for its specific form (fresh, dried, powdered, or juiced), the digestive system begins its absorption and distribution of the powerful compounds such as the antioxidants, enzymes, oils, and polyphenols to every area of the body. Being delivered directly to the site of the cancerous growth, ginger's cancer-fighting compounds begin a cell-ravaging crusade that seeks and destroys cancerous cells while promoting the growth of healthy cells surrounding them. Ginger's unique blend of oils, nutrients, and phytochemicals also inhibits inflammation to reduce joint pain, regulates hormone and blood sugar levels to help reduce nausea, and improves digestive system functioning to minimize vomiting. The circulatory system and metabolism also benefit from ginger, helping to improve the energy levels and mental functioning of the chemotherapy patient.

55. HELPS REVERSE LIVER DAMAGE

Liver damage is considered to be any disturbance of liver functioning, contributing to or causing illnesses related to the liver. While liver damage can be done to a minor or excessive extent, only patients dealing with a liver that has endured damage to 75 percent of the structure are considered to be suffering from liver disease; it is at this 75 percent threshold that symptoms and conditions begin to arise. A staggering number of contributing factors can wreak havoc on the liver's health and functioning, including inflammation of liver cells, obstructed bile flow, compromised blood flow, tissue damage, viral infections, or damage done by toxins, prescriptions, and even over-the-counter medications. Because this organ is absolutely essential in manufacturing, processing, utilizing, and ridding the body of important nutrients, hormones, and fluids, the liver should be cared for and maintained in order to ensure optimal health. Long before liver disease damage can minimize functioning and be a potential concern for the future health of the organ and its related systems.

Through the consumption of a clean diet that includes ginger, anyone can improve their liver's functioning and reverse damage that may have occurred. With a diet clear of excessive fats, sugars, sodium, and toxins that can degrade the liver and require hard-working effort on the liver's part, the first step to liver repair can be achieved. After all, less strain and demand on the liver means more of the organ's effort can be directed toward its repair. Luckily, ginger has a unique, naturally occurring oil called 6-gingerol that has been identified as one of the most effective compounds for preventing buildup of fats in the liver, which helps minimize the workload and improve the liver's optimal functioning. Ginger also provides unique antioxidant properties along with specialized detoxifying enzymes, which help to support the liver's functioning while also improving the condition of the organ itself.

56. DETOXIFIES THE LIVER

The liver is the detoxification center for the entire body, responsible for cleansing the blood, nutrients, and waste, and removing unnecessary, excess, or toxic substances from the body. Unfortunately, this specialized organ that helps filter and cleanse the body can become overly taxed through excessive use, resulting from a number of situations such as alcohol consumption, poor dietary habits, or malnutrition. A less-than-optimal liver can lead to diminished functioning of any of the body's organs or systems, and a likely development of signs and symptoms such as fatigue, nausea, constipation, or even yellowing of the eyes and skin within a short period of time. Because of the crucial role the liver plays in keeping the body clear of harmful toxins; maintaining stabilized blood sugar, hormone, and cholesterol levels; and promoting proper metabolism of nutrients in the process of energy production, it is easy to see why the liver must be free of challenges or illness in order to ensure optimal overall functioning.

Ginger has a variety of natural phytochemicals, oils, and compounds such as gingerol and shogaol that promote enzymatic reactions throughout the body, so it's no surprise that those same phytochemicals help the body in the process of xenobiotic detoxification (a metabolic detoxification or natural processing of nutrients performed within the body) that rids the liver of harmful, unwanted toxins. This special detoxification process uses ginger's compounds to purge excess fat build-up in the liver, remove waste from the bloodstream and liver, and burn toxins that would otherwise be shuttled to the liver for processing and removal. With the decreased workload on the liver, the organ's natural process of cell regeneration helps to begin and sustain a healthy detoxification. With ginger's ability to improve nutrient absorption, along with its natural support of the circulatory and metabolic systems, both heavily involved with the detoxification processes, it's no wonder that ginger can be a healthy addition to any detoxification plan focused on the liver.

57. PREVENTS ULCERS

Ulcers—holes and/or breaks in the protective lining of the upper part of the small intestine (also known as the duodenum), the stomach, or the esophagus—are becoming a common condition that strikes one out of every ten Americans. While these uncomfortable areas of erosion in the lining of the digestive canals take significant time to develop, the considerable degradation that can occur during that time can be severe. Their development can be caused by a combination of a number of factors, including smoking, alcohol consumption, bacterial infections, excessive stomach acid secretions, and over-the-counter painkillers (such as acetaminophen). While over-the-counter and prescription medications intended to reduce the erosive stomach acid thought to be to blame for ulcers may be effective initially, there is the possibility of serious side effects such as adversely affected pH balance or minimized natural enzyme production by the body, which is why there are warnings against the long-term use of these products.

Ginger has been shown to be an effective, all-natural treatment method for repairing ulcers and preventing their development in the future. In one study published in the *Indian Journal of Pharmacological Science* in 2009 that investigated the effectiveness of ginger in stomach discomfort, researchers were able to observe ginger's unique oils inhibit the growth of a specific bacteria, *Helicobacter pylori* (*H. pylori*), that is often associated with the development of peptic ulcers that form within the digestive system. With the same comparable dose of the 1 teaspoon of freshly grated ginger that helps to fight the *H. pylori* bacteria, ulcer sufferers can also benefit from stabilized stomach acid levels, reduced inflammation, improved digestion, more efficient metabolism, and better blood flow, all of which directly promote optimal health within the digestive system and have shown to prevent ulcers effectively and naturally.

58. DETOXIFIES THE INTESTINES

With their muscular tubes that are able to shuttle food down, around, and out of the body, the large and small intestines are perfectly poised for digestive success. Throughout the digestive process, these intestines are responsible for extracting as much water content and nutrients from the food as possible; those nutrients will then be absorbed and utilized throughout the body in various processes. The specialized glands related to the digestive processes, as well as the enzymatic reactions of the chemicals excreted by these intestines, allow for the food consumed to be absorbed, stored, and utilized for any and all functions and processes going on in the body.

But the intestines do so much more than digest food. Housing a startling percentage of the body's immune system, the intestines are the lifeline to health. By maintaining clean intestines free and clear of debris and toxins, the health of the digestive system and every other system in its network can be preserved.

With every consumed particle passing through these intestines, it's easy to see how particles, debris, and toxins can be caught in the folds or crevasses; understanding that these bits can be left behind as food passes can make it easier to understand how the need for detoxification can develop over time. With the use of ginger, the detoxification process can be a natural, effective process that also promotes healing, prevents illness, and optimizes the functioning and health of each and every one of the body's systems. Ginger directly provides the intestines with antioxidants, antimicrobial agents, bad-bacteria-fighting enzymes, and intestine-cleansing fiber, and also provides the added benefits of optimized blood flow, maximum nutrient absorption, and regulated hormone balance, all of which make ginger one of the best detoxification agents available to the intestines.

59. MINIMIZES INFLAMMATION OF THE COLON

Inflammation, the immune system's response to infection or irritation at any site, can occur within any tissue in the body. When inflammation occurs in a site that is visible to the eye, redness, swelling, and irritation are the most obvious symptoms. But inflammation can be difficult to detect with internal organs like the colon, simply because it is impossible to see any obvious signs of irritation or inflammation.

With a variety of conditions such as ulcerative colitis, Crohn's disease, and irritable bowel diseases and syndromes stemming from inflammation within the colon, the importance of preventing and treating the causes and contributing factors to inflammation at this site is a must! Without treatment, these conditions can result in painful digestive symptoms that range from severe diarrhea, pain, fatigue, and weight loss, to the development of sores and ulcers within the stomach lining to life-threatening complications. Fortunately, the introduction of ginger into a treatment regimen can reduce the colon's inflammation and improve the rate and success of repair.

Ginger's powerful anti-inflammatory compounds, gingerol and shogaol, combine to effectively calm inflammation directly at the site of irritation. These compounds are extremely effective when dealing with the colon due to their natural abilities to deliver essential nutrients needed for repair, antimicrobial agents that combat the cause of the irritation, and pain-relieving analgesic compounds that can deliver pain relief to the site. Ginger's blood-cleansing and health-promoting phytochemicals are also able to help improve the rate of white blood cell production and optimize cell regeneration, which work wonders on colon conditions by optimizing the effectiveness of the body's natural detoxification process, minimizing inflammation of the colon that can lead to an increase in trapped undigested or partially digested particles, and relieving pain and discomfort resulting from colon inflammation . . . naturally!

60. RELIEVES CONSTIPATION

Constipation is a condition characterized by the inability to pass waste in bowel movements regularly or without straining. Constipation can result from a number of causes ranging from a poor diet, excessive stress, or inadequate exercise, to certain pre-existing conditions (such as pregnancy) or even medications. Whatever the reason, dealing with constipation can be a frustrating and debilitating endeavor that is only further complicated by the feeling that there is no end in sight. When constipation lasts for prolonged periods of time, or occurs frequently, the results of stagnant waste being trapped in the intestine can inhibit the body's natural processes of nutrient absorption, allow toxins to seep into the intestines and throughout the body, minimize immunity, and even pollute the bloodstream. With a number of prescription constipation aids and over-the-counter treatment options available, the options for "getting things moving" can be overwhelming, but it's important to understand that not all of these constipation aids are effective. Many contain powerful synthetic stimulants, and some can produce dangerous side effects such as dehydration, cognitive dysfunction, or even systemic issues and blockages that require surgery for correction, all of which far outweigh the discomfort of constipation.

With an all-natural combination of ginger, a constipation sufferer can find relief quickly, safely, and without worrying about dangerous or uncomfortable side effects. The phytochemicals found in ginger directly promote the digestive system's functioning and metabolism, which get things moving. Ginger also improves muscle action within the intestines, colon, and rectum, and increases the secretion of digestive enzymes and lubricating mucus, all of which help to form stools and move them through the proper passages with ease. By helping to relieve toxin buildup in the bowels and bloodstream as a result of stagnant stools, ginger is able to keep the body clear of infection until things return to "regular."

61. PREVENTS GAS

Resulting from poor diet, medications, or even stress, gas can produce bloating, excessive flatulence or burping, and excruciating pain in the abdominal area. The good news is that, with simple preventative and treatment options, you can avoid the need for over-the-counter treatment options that pose dangerous health risks or that can leave you dealing with additional side effects. Tried and true remedies that focus on treating the cause of the gas, while also preventing the future occurrences of excessive gas development, are not only more effective than their synthetic counterparts, but can also provide the body with additional support, safely and naturally.

One of the most commonly used treatments for gas is ginger. Widely used throughout Asia for thousands of years, ginger has been one of the most effective treatments for digestive issues and complications, including gas. Known for being a carminative, an herb or application that helps expel gas, ginger's unique oils and phytochemicals attack the issue head-on and actually encourage the specific enzymatic reactions that become disrupted and contribute to the formation of gas. Stimulating digestion and the metabolism, ginger also helps to move disruptive foods through the digestive system quickly in order to prevent the development of gas. With naturally antiseptic and anti-inflammatory properties, ginger's support also inhibits the development of conditions such as indigestion, constipation, or inadequate nutrient absorption, which can quickly develop gas as a symptom. Promoting health while preventing gas, ginger is one of the most promising safe and effective treatment options available.

62. PROMOTES REGULARITY

Physicians have long struggled to determine what constitutes "regularity" concerning bowel movements, how to promote regularity, and how to alleviate the common conditions that can interfere with regularity. While not all physicians agree, the most widely accepted parameters for being "regular" fall within the range of three bowel movements per day to three movements per week. Irregularity is understood to be fewer than three bowel movements per week, and most patients who experience irregularity also report consistent bloating and abdominal discomfort, chronic fatigue, frequent illness, and physical conditions such as hemorrhoids and anal fissures (tears around the rectum). Luckily, there is a natural treatment option available that can promote regularity effectively: ginger!

With the addition of ginger, you can achieve regularity, maintain regularity, and avoid the conditions and symptoms that result from a dysfunctional digestive system. While ginger can be useful in preventing constipation, ginger's multiple phytochemicals, enzymes, and oils, along with its rich antioxidants and anti-inflammatory compounds, combine to promote regularity on a systemic level by not only improving digestion and minimizing common conditions related to irregularity, but improving the health and functioning of all of the body's systems related to regularity as well! Promoting optimal metabolic functioning, improving the secretion of digestive enzymes, and supporting the glands responsible for the release of lubricating mucus in the intestines, ginger can help move stools efficiently. Helping to remove toxins that may have accumulated through the extended stay of stools awaiting exit, ginger is also able to prevent illness and conditions, further improved with its provisions of antimicrobial, antiseptic, antibacterial properties. With the added benefit of ginger's vitamins, minerals, amino acids, enzymes, and fiber, the restoration of regularity is accompanied by the improved functioning of every one of the body's systems!

63. MINIMIZES MENSTRUAL PAIN

Menstrual pain, also known as dysmenorrhea, is characterized by abdominal pain, back pain, cramping, and fatigue. This is a common condition, with an estimated 85 percent of women experiencing minor to severe discomfort around the time of menstruation. While many women endure these symptoms to a degree and duration that allows for undisrupted daily life to continue, a growing number of women are reporting extreme discomfort for longer durations of time that exceed the previous estimated "average" of 3–5 days. In an effort to identify the most effective form of pain relief for women experiencing severe menstrual pain symptoms, researchers conducted a double-blind study comparing a placebo, ibuprofen, and ginger. The results were astounding!

The 2013 study, published in the *Journal of Alternative and Complementary Medicine*, concluded that the group of women (50 out of the 150 total participants) who were provided with 250 mg of powdered ginger four times daily reported less menstrual pain and faster recovery time than the group who were provided with 400 mg of ibuprofen four times daily. With natural anti-inflammatory properties in ginger's oils, enzymes, and phytochemicals that are able to seek and relieve concentrated areas of inflammation in the body, ginger is not only able to alleviate inflammation that can cause discomfort, but also relieve pain through its provisions of natural analgesic compounds provided by the enzymes and oils. With its ability to improve iron absorption in the bloodstream, maintain optimal hormone levels, and promote proper metabolic and digestive functioning, ginger is also able to minimize fatigue, mood swings, and bloating. Ginger may be the best possible go-to menstrual pain reliever that provides safe, effective, all-natural relief!

64. ACTS AS A NATURAL APHRODISIAC

Today's medical advances have led to an overwhelming number of sexual health aides designed to improve desire, increase sensitivity, and extend endurance, with the goal being to enhance the sexual experience. Like most synthetic treatments, though, the risks of side effects that can result from taking these medications is great, with discomfort, pain, and even death being possibilities. However, for thousands of years, ancient cultures have utilized ginger for a wide variety of treatments—including sexual stimulation. Today, ginger is making a comeback to take hold as the age-old, tried and tested, scientifically proven, all-natural, extremely effective aphrodisiac that can improve sexual health and better the sexual experience . . . for men *and* women.

The spicy reputation of ginger is one of the most important elements of this formula. The ginger root's provisions of naturally occurring oils, enzymes, and nutrients such as gingerol, shogaol, and the assortment of vitamins and minerals that combine to stimulate the senses do so by activating the nervous system, raising the heart rate, and improving circulation. These specific reactions in the body mimic how the body feels in response to sexual stimulation and work to trigger an arousal, both physically and psychologically. In addition, ginger may also contribute to male and female fertility. One 2010 study performed by the veterinary pharmacology department of the Shiraz University of Medical Sciences that explored the sexual effects of ginger powder on the fertility of rats observed "increased sperm motility and viability" in those who had received the ginger doses, concluding that ginger invigorates the reproductive organs. While regular ingestion of a small amount of ginger will not elicit a sexual response, the spicy root can improve the many systems of the body related to sexual health, improving the body's natural sexual response in appropriate situations; the thermogenic effect in the body created by ginger's oils and enzymes like gingerol can, in fact, mimic the body's sexual response in terms of an increased heart rate, increased body temperature, etc.

65. INFUSES PULLING OIL FOR IMPROVED EFFECTIVENESS

"Pulling" is an age-old method long used by civilizations and cultures around the world to rid the body of toxins. While the original method focuses on only extended swishing of oil in the mouth, the addition of ginger has shown promise in removing toxins from the body by delivering protective antioxidants, and protecting the entire body from dangerous changes in the blood and within the cells by improving immunity and maintaining cell health. This Ginger-Infused Pulling Oil tastes great, relieves bad breath, and improves your overall health, and the process of pulling can be assimilated into any morning routine! With the added benefits of whiter teeth, healthier teeth and gums, and a drastic reduction in germs, bacteria, and viruses that can wreak havoc on the mouth, this simple combination of coconut oil and ginger can be one of the most beneficial 20-minute tasks you do throughout the day . . . not only for wellness, but for your quality of life, too!

TO MAKE 3–5 APPLICATIONS OF THE GINGER-INFUSED PULLING OIL, USE:

½ tablespoon powdered ginger
¼ cup liquid coconut oil

1. Combine ginger and coconut oil in an 8-ounce glass or jar, and shake vigorously to combine well.
2. Sip approximately 1–2 oz. of the mixture, then swish the mixture around the mouth and through the teeth for 10–20 minutes.
3. Spit the mixture (do not swallow!) and rinse the mouth thoroughly with water.

Recommendations for use: For best results, this method should be used 5–7 days per week. Results should be noticeable within 1–3 uses. Store remaining Pulling Oil in the glass jar used to combine in Step 1, sealed tightly and stored in a cool, dark place. Do not refrigerate. Use within 5 days of mixing.

KEEP IT UP!

This pulling method can be tiring for the first few trials; the goal is to continue the swishing process (without swallowing the oil!) for a period of no less than 20 minutes. While a few minutes will provide benefits, the maximum benefits of pulling result after bacteria and microbes have been released from the oral areas after 20 minutes of vigorous swishing. Muscles of the mouth will increase in ability relating to stamina, allowing for longer "pulling" time periods to be sustained with ease over time.

PART II

BEAUTY

Chapter 3

SKIN CARE

When it comes to skin care, there is no doubt that natural products are the best bet for safe and effective results. While there are a staggering number of synthetic products available, many even claiming to be "all-natural" or touting claims that they include "all-natural ingredients," these products are rarely comprised of ingredients free of chemicals and additives, and some of them may even harm your skin. The good news is that you need look no further than the fabulous ginger root if you're looking for healthy products that promote healing, rejuvenation, and refreshing results.

Packed with an abundance of naturally occurring oils, enzymes, phytochemicals, and nutrients that combine to promote the natural beauty of your skin, ginger is able to work wonders in almost every area of skin care safely, naturally, and effectively! Throughout this chapter, you'll learn all you need to know about the most common skin-care needs, as well as how ginger can be used to improve, revive, and heal skin conditions, appearances, and health. The best part is that, with the ingredients used in these do-it-yourself homemade remedies, the skin gets nutrient-rich care for real results without dangerous side effects or reactions. All-natural, health-promoting, effective, and safe, this spicy little root is about to change your skin for the better!

66. CLEARS ACNE

Physicians have determined that a combination of factors including age, hormone levels, genetics, anxiety and stress levels, and hot or humid climates can all contribute to the development of acne. Even oil-based makeup, poor hygiene practices, and oily hair can be to blame for acne outbreaks. While seemingly different, these factors all involve a disruption in the oil production of the sebaceous glands and their release of those oils along tiny hair follicles on your face, back, chest, shoulders, neck, and arms. Once this process has been disrupted, the oils can get trapped beneath the skin, breeding bacteria and irritation, resulting in the development of acne.

Ginger, when used in the following Acne-Clearing Mask, rescues acne sufferers with its naturally occurring oils, enzymes, and phytochemicals found in the natural provisions of vitamins A, C, and E that fight acne-causing bacteria, prevent inflammation and irritation, and deliver soothing skin-healing properties directly to the site of breakouts. Whether the outbreak is mild, moderate, or severe, the addition of ginger's oils to your beauty routine can benefit your skin and banish breakouts!

TO MAKE 1 APPLICATION OF THE ACNE-CLEARING MASK, USE:

¼ cup strawberries

1 tablespoon grated ginger

1 teaspoon lemon juice

1. Mash strawberries until completely pulped, then combine strawberries, ginger, and lemon juice in a blender and blend on high until thoroughly combined.
2. Apply the mixture to the face liberally, focusing on the most problem-prone areas of the skin. Allow mask to remain on skin for 15–20 minutes.
3. Rinse mask from skin thoroughly using a washcloth soaked with warm water by applying the washcloth to the skin's surface for approximately one minute before using gentle circular motions to cleanse the skin's surface.

Recommendations for use: For best results, this treatment should be used for a time period of 15–20 minutes, 5–7 days per week. Results should be noticeable within 1–3 weeks.

67. TONES SKIN

With age, sun exposure, environmental conditions, and certain illnesses or specific skin conditions, the skin on the face and throughout the body can become unevenly toned. Ginger provides the skin with an abundance of nutrients and phytochemicals like resveratrol, as well as enzymes that not only help to repair skin with the building of elastin and collagen, but encourage the regeneration of skin cells free of discoloration. With antioxidants that help to prevent damage, ginger adds beauty and health benefits to unevenly toned skin. For a great mask that can be used on the face or any part of the body with uneven skin tone, simply use the following Toning Mask that includes ginger for antioxidants and skin-repairing elements, green tea for antioxidants and circulation-stimulating benefits, and coconut oil to ensure smooth, moisturized skin:

1. Remove green tea leaves from cooled, steeped tea bag.
2. Combine tea leaves, powdered ginger, and coconut oil, and mix until thoroughly combined.
3. Apply the mixture to the unevenly toned skin liberally, focusing on the most problem-prone areas of the skin and allow mask to remain on skin for 15–20 minutes.
4. Rinse mask from skin thoroughly using a washcloth soaked with warm water by applying the washcloth to the skin's surface for approximately one minute before using gentle circular motions to cleanse the skin's surface.

Recommendations for use: For best results, this treatment should be used for a time period of 15–20 minutes, 5–7 days per week. Results should be noticeable within 2 weeks.

TO MAKE 1 APPLICATION OF THE TONING MASK, USE:

1 tablespoon cooled green tea leaves
  (from steeped tea bag)
1 tablespoon powdered ginger
2 tablespoons coconut oil

68. REDUCES APPEARANCE OF SCARS

Scars are unsightly appearances on the surface of the skin that can vary in size and color, characteristic of skin being biologically repaired following a disruption, agitation, or trauma to the skin's surface. Many products are available that claim to reduce the appearance of scars, but most contain harsh ingredients that can leave the treated area irritated with the scar remaining. Ginger, on the other hand, provides the skin with a number of naturally occurring phytochemicals that help to reverse the hypopigmentation and hyperpigmentation that occur within the skin as scar tissue develops during the healing process; these oils and enzymes, known as gingerol and shogaol, not only combat illness and infection during healing, but also improve the body's natural regeneration through the efficient production of new skin cells while delivering antioxidant and anti-inflammatory benefits to the site of new skin cell production. Further supporting the repair of the skin's surface are the gentle collagen- and elastin-building proteins and enzymes found in ginger, helping to rejuvenate and repair skin's cells with the healthy composition and elasticity of youthful skin. By adding the powerful ginger root to a combination of additional skin-protecting ingredients, such as carrot juice and coconut oil, you can create a repairing salve suitable for scars anywhere on the skin.

TO MAKE 1 APPLICATION OF SCAR-HEALING SALVE, USE:

2 tablespoons carrot juice

1 tablespoon freshly juiced ginger

½ cup coconut oil

1. Combine carrot juice, ginger, and coconut oil in a blender. Blend at high speed until thoroughly combined, or about 1–2 minutes.
2. Apply the mixture liberally to the scarred skin, focusing on the most problem-prone areas, and allow mixture to remain on skin for 15–20 minutes.
3. Rinse mixture from skin thoroughly using a washcloth soaked with warm water by applying the washcloth to the skin's surface for approximately one minute before using gentle circular motions to cleanse the skin's surface.

Recommendations for use: For best results, this treatment should be used for a time period of 15–20 minutes, 3–5 times per day. Results should be noticeable within 4–8 weeks.

69. SOOTHES SUNBURNS

In the short periods of time that skin is left vulnerable to the sun's rays, even after applying sunscreen or sunblock, the damage to the skin's cells can result in hazardous or even deadly conditions! It is absolutely imperative to treat those sunburned areas of the skin immediately in order to safeguard the skin's cells and tissues from cancerous changes that can quickly affect cells, tissues, and systems throughout the body. Ginger is one of the best treatments for sunburned skin, providing unique oils like gingerol and shogaol, as well as powerful antioxidants like vitamins A, C, and E that have been shown to prevent the cancerous changes in skin's cells. This root can be combined with vitamin E oil for advanced skin-repairing benefits, and aloe vera with moisturizing, antioxidant, and additional skin-reparative properties to create this Soothing Balm that will support the healing process and protect the skin from past and future damage.

1. Combine aloe vera, ginger, and vitamin E oil in a blender, and blend on high speed until thoroughly combined, or about 1–2 minutes.

2. Apply the mixture to the affected skin liberally and allow balm to remain on skin until fully absorbed. Each application should be permitted to stay on the skin without interference for 15–20 minutes, or until fully absorbed, before dressing or covering with cloth of any kind (if required).

3. If the application needs to be removed prior to being completely absorbed, gently wipe away excess balm from the skin using a dry or warm, damp washcloth by applying the washcloth to the skin's surface and using gentle circular motions to cleanse the skin's surface with minimal agitation.

Recommendations for use: For best results, this treatment should be used as often as necessary to provide relief.

TO MAKE 1 APPLICATION OF THE SOOTHING BALM, USE:

½ cup aloe vera gel

2 tablespoon powdered ginger

5 drops vitamin E oil

70. INFUSES MASSAGE OIL WITH HEALING BENEFITS

Massage oils can be simple aromatic additions to any foot rub, massage, or scrub that increases the sensuality, stimulation, and satisfaction of those experiences. But, while many would consider those pleasurable benefits to be enough, ginger can add an aromatic element to any massage oil, while also effectively enhancing the experience of massage through an abundance of phytonutrients such as antioxidants, anti-inflammatory properties, and a wide variety of vitamins and minerals that combine to create an incredibly sensual experience with a multitude of health benefits as well. Researchers have studied the root and determined that ginger truly is able to stimulate the senses, improve circulation, increase sensitivity, and increase the body's temperature, helping to heighten the physical experience of a massage with biological and topical reactions that create an intensified massage experience. When applied directly to the skin, ginger's oils can intensify a massage oil's effects exponentially. Without the fear of harmful side effects that can be caused by harsh synthetic additives contained in over-the-counter massage oils, a simple combination of sweet, spicy, and soothing natural ingredients can take your massage experience to the next level, safely and naturally. With the spiciness of ginger, the sweet aroma of pineapple, and the soothing sensation of coconut oil added to the following Ginger-Infused Massage Oil, your massage can be your best yet, with benefits for your mind, body, and soul.

TO MAKE 1 APPLICATION OF GINGER-INFUSED MASSAGE OIL:

1 cup coconut oil
4 tablespoons fresh pineapple juice
2 tablespoons fresh ginger juice

1. In a blender, combine coconut oil, pineapple juice, and ginger juice, and blend on high speed for 1–2 minutes, or until ingredients are thoroughly combined.
2. Use liberally while massaging any area of the body.

Recommendations for use: If making in advance, store in a sealed container in a cool, dark place for up to 3 days. To reconstitute, blend as instructed in Step 1.

71. HEALS CRACKED SKIN ON HEELS

Not surprisingly, one of the most neglected areas of the body is the heel. With the pressure and friction on your heels that can occur just as a result of daily wear and tear, the skin on the heels can quickly become dry, cracked, and irritated. Fortunately, a Ginger Foot Scrub is all you need to resolve this common condition. With the skin-repairing phytochemicals, rejuvenating nutrients, and collagen- and elastin-promoting oils and enzymes found in ginger, this scrub can rejuvenate the skin on your heels in no time. Combined with a reparative combination of circulation-stimulating green tea, granulated sugar to help exfoliate dead skin, and rich oils that penetrate the skin with moisturizing benefits, the antioxidant-rich ginger found in this foot soak that doubles as a scrub is the perfect prescription for an effective all-natural heel healing solution!

TO MAKE 1 APPLICATION OF THE GINGER FOOT SCRUB, USE:

3 tablespoons powdered ginger

½ cup coconut oil

2 cups green tea, prepared and cooled to lukewarm temperature

2 cups granulated sugar

1. In a soaking tub just large enough for the feet, combine the ginger, oil, and green tea. Soak your feet in the solution for about 10–15 minutes, or until skin is softened.

2. Add sugar to the solution. Scooping a handful of the solution into the hands, proceed to scrub the heels with the sugar by massaging the granulated solution into the skin.

3. Continue the scrubbing process as necessary until skin feels softened, then rinse.

Recommendations for use: For best results, this treatment should be used for a time period of 15–30 minutes, 5–7 days per week. Results should be noticeable within 1–2 applications.

KEEP YOUR HEELS SILKY SMOOTH

To really ensure that your heels are silky smooth, once you rinse off the scrub, moisturize them with the Moisturizing Mask found in the following entry.

72. MOISTURIZES SKIN

With dry, cold weather conditions, physical reactions to certain foods, chronic disorders, and/or a myriad of situations that compromise the natural balance of the skin's condition, skin on the face and throughout the body can become dry. If you look in any store, you'll find a dizzying number of products available that promise to relieve dry skin, provide skin with natural healing elements, and deliver the naturally beautiful skin you seek. The only problem is that these products often contain synthetic, irritating, or abrasive components that may lead to side effects, irritation, or even increased dryness. Luckily, ginger can resolve dry skin issues naturally by providing your skin with vitamins like A, C, and E; minerals like calcium and magnesium; unique ginger oils and enzymes like gingerol and shogaol; and multiple amino acids that combine to support the structures and processes that are responsible for skin's health like the sebaceous glands and skin cells within every layer of the skin. In addition, ginger can help prevent the irritating issues that contribute to dryness such as infections, inflammation, oil buildup, and immune system dysfunctions, effectively and safely!

TO MAKE 1 APPLICATION OF THE MOISTURIZING MASK, USE:

½ cup yogurt

3 tablespoons honey

2 tablespoons juiced ginger

1. Combine yogurt, honey, and ginger juice in an 8-ounce jar with a tight-fitting lid. Mix at medium speed with a fork or whisk for 1–2 minutes, or until ingredients are thoroughly combined.

2. Apply the mixture to the skin liberally with your hands, focusing on the most problem-prone areas, and allow mask to remain on skin for 15–20 minutes.

3. Rinse mask from skin thoroughly using a washcloth soaked with warm water by applying the washcloth to the skin's surface for approximately one minute before using gentle circular motions to cleanse the skin's surface.

Recommendations for use: For best results, this treatment should be used for a time period of 15–20 minutes, 5–7 days per week. Results should be noticeable within 1–2 weeks.

73. PROMOTES RADIANT SKIN

Free of blemishes, unsightly dark spots, irritation, and redness, radiant skin exudes a healthy glow that just can't be bought. While store-bought creams and potions promise to deliver beautiful, healthy skin, they often fall short for one very important reason: radiant skin results from optimal health on the inside, not just on the skin's surface. When your body is well nourished, functioning at its best, and maintains an optimal level of health in all of its systems, the results are seen and felt in every area of the body . . . especially the skin.

With the addition of ginger to your daily diet, you can promote your skin's health easily and naturally. With ample amounts of nutrients like beta-carotene, B vitamins, vitamins C and E, iron, and magnesium, all combining to promote circulation, improve metabolic functioning, support the regeneration of cells, and protect the cells against free radical damage, ginger is able to promote a healthy, radiant glow from the inside out! Add topical applications of ginger like this Radiant Skin Mask to a daily consumption of the spicy root, and your skin is sure to benefit from a variety of properties that combine to create the perfect inner balance for outer beauty!

TO MAKE 1 APPLICATION OF THE RADIANT SKIN MASK, USE:

2 tablespoons powdered ginger

2 tablespoons honey

2 tablespoons lemon juice

1 teaspoon apple cider vinegar

1. Combine ginger, honey, lemon juice, and apple cider vinegar in a shallow dish and whisk vigorously for approximately 1 minute, or until ingredients are thoroughly combined.

2. Apply the mixture to the face or body liberally, focusing on the most problem-prone areas, and allow mask to remain on the skin for 15–20 minutes.

3. Rinse mask from skin thoroughly using a washcloth soaked with warm water by applying the washcloth to the skin's surface for approximately one minute before using gentle circular motions to cleanse the skin's surface.

Recommendations for use: For best results, this treatment should be used for a time period of 15–20 minutes, 5–7 days per week. Results should be noticeable within 1–2 weeks.

74. OPTIMIZES THE DETOXIFYING ATTRIBUTES OF A BODY SOAK

Toxins, environmental factors, and waste debris can not only wreak havoc on the body, bloodstream, and brain, but on the skin, eyes, hair, nails, and numerous systems throughout the body. Fortunately, ginger provides a number of powerful naturally occurring phytochemicals such as gingerol that help relieve the body of harmful chemicals, toxins, and carcinogenic compounds that can collect in the body from the diet, the environment, and the dysfunction of healthy processes that are intended to rid the body of such waste. Ginger is also able to improve the functioning of the detoxifying powerhouse, the liver, by providing supportive oils, enzymes, and nutrients that combine to keep the body and brain running optimally and protected against harmful changes that can occur within cells, tissues, organs, and systems. In addition to its benefits when consumed in its many forms, the addition of ginger to this Detoxifying Soak increases its effectiveness exponentially. With the ability to extract toxins, fight free radicals, provide nutrients, and support system functioning of all sorts, this gingery soak is the perfect detoxifying, health-improving resolution!

TO MAKE 1 APPLICATION OF THE DETOXIFYING SOAK, USE:

½ cup Epsom salts

½ cup sea salt

½ cup baking soda

2 cups apple cider vinegar

¼ cup freshly grated ginger

1. In an 8-ounce Mason jar with a tight-fitting lid, combine all ingredients, secure lid, and shake well to combine thoroughly.
2. As warm or hot water fills a bathtub, gradually add the contents of the jar, allowing the contents to dissolve and disperse throughout the water.
3. Soak in the treated water for 20–45 minutes, then rinse and towel dry as usual.

Recommendations for use: For best results, this treatment should be used for a time period of 20–45 minutes, 1–3 days per week.

75. RELIEVES DRY SKIN

When you suffer from dry skin, it can seem counterproductive to adopt a beauty regimen that involves scrubbing or exfoliating, simply because of the possibility that the process could lead to even more dryness. However, an exfoliating scrub actually removes the dead layers of skin that can lead to dry, itchy, irritated skin conditions, and the addition of a moisturizing component improves the condition of dry skin even more. The essential part of this Skin-Replenishing Body Scrub is the addition of ginger, which not only helps to safeguard skin against damaging components such as environmental factors or cellular oxidation caused by free radicals that can lead to minor to severe conditions resulting in the development of dry skin, but also delivers a unique blend of nutrients like moisturizing oils, replenishing vitamins and minerals, and an abundance of protective antioxidants and anti-inflammatory compounds that promote skin health.

TO MAKE 1–3 APPLICATIONS OF THE SKIN-REPLENISHING BODY SCRUB, USE:

¼ cup coconut oil

1 tablespoon chopped ginger

¼ cup almond oil

¾ cup granulated sugar

¼ cup coarse kosher salt

1–4 drops essential oil (lavender, rose, lemongrass, etc.)

1. Heat coconut oil and ginger in a small saucepan over low heat for 5–10 minutes, or until fragrant.
2. Remove from heat, add almond oil, and stir to combine, setting aside to cool for 30–60 minutes. Transfer cooled mixture to a 16-ounce Mason jar with a tight-fitting lid.
3. Add sugar and salt, along with essential oils.
4. While showering or bathing, gently apply the scrub to the skin with a washcloth using circular motions. Rinse, and towel dry as usual.

Recommendations for use: For best results, this scrub should be used 2–4 days per week. Results should be noticeable within 1–3 uses. Store remaining scrub in sealed Mason jar in a cool, dark place (not refrigerated) for no more than 5–7 days.

76. DIMINISHES WRINKLES

The desire for wrinkle-free skin is one that is shared by people around the world, and has been for centuries. New medical procedures promise to banish fine lines and wrinkles from the face with a simple injection, application, or treatment, but do so with the use of harsh chemicals that can lead to serious side effects, complications, and even disfigurement. Luckily, there are a few all-natural ingredients that can be combined to deliver the same results safely, naturally, and with little cost. The star ingredient of this treatment is none other than ginger!

Providing the skin with unique oils and enzymes such as shogaol and gingerol, as well as vitamins A, C, and E, and a multitude of minerals such as iron and magnesium that stimulate circulation, improve collagen and elastin production, and provide skin cells with antioxidant benefits, ginger is able to safeguard the skin's health while also improving its appearance. With the addition of natural ingredients, like pineapple juice, egg whites, and honey, you can create an easy and inexpensive Anti-Wrinkle Mask that's not only effective, but safe enough to use every single day!

TO MAKE 1 APPLICATION OF THE ANTI-WRINKLE MASK, USE:

2 tablespoons pineapple juice

2 tablespoons grated ginger

1 egg white, beaten

1 teaspoon honey

1. Combine pineapple juice, ginger, egg white, and honey in a blender, and blend on medium to high for 1–2 minutes, or until ingredients are thoroughly combined.

2. Apply the mixture to the face liberally and gently with fingertips in circular motions, focusing on the most wrinkle-prone areas of the skin, then allow mask to remain on skin for 15–20 minutes.

3. Rinse mask from skin thoroughly using a washcloth soaked with warm water by applying the washcloth to the skin's surface for approximately one minute before using gentle circular motions to cleanse the skin's surface.

Recommendations for use: For best results, this treatment should be used for a time period of 15–20 minutes, 7 days per week. Results should be noticeable within 2–6 weeks.

77. PROMOTES YOUTHFUL-LOOKING SKIN

Anti-aging products account for a whopping ten billion dollars of the annual total generated by the skin-care industry. Fortunately, in order to achieve the goals of reduced fine lines and wrinkles, even skin tone, and a clean and clear complexion, you need look no further than the all-natural ginger root!

Through its provisions of vitamins, minerals, antioxidants, and unique oils and enzymes, ginger promotes the skin's regeneration of healthy skin cells, production of skin-firming collagen and elastin, and bacteria- and germ-free conditioning for a clear and healthy complexion. Add to these benefits a glow that can only come from improved circulation and maximum nutrient absorption, and it's easy to see why ginger may just be the perfect anti-aging ingredient.

This Anti-Aging Mask promotes a more youthful appearance on the outside while optimizing health on the inside. With ginger, you can supply your skin with all of the natural anti-aging properties it needs!

TO MAKE 1 APPLICATION OF THE ANTI-AGING MASK, USE:

2 tablespoons fresh carrot juice

2 tablespoons pineapple juice

2 tablespoons powdered ginger

2 tablespoons aloe vera gel

1 teaspoon lemon juice

2 tablespoons coconut oil

1. Combine carrot juice, pineapple juice, powdered ginger, aloe vera gel, lemon juice, and coconut oil in a blender, and blend at medium to high speed until all ingredients are thoroughly combined.
2. Apply the mixture to the face liberally with fingertips using circular motions, evenly distributing the mixture over the entire skin's surface, and allow mask to remain on skin for 15–20 minutes.
3. Rinse mask from skin thoroughly using a washcloth soaked with warm water by applying the washcloth to the skin's surface for approximately one minute before using gentle circular motions to cleanse the skin's surface.

Recommendations for use: For best results, this treatment should be used for a time period of 15–20 minutes, 5–7 days per week. Results should be noticeable within 2–4 weeks.

78. REPAIRS SKIN DISCOLORATION

With a number of factors that contribute to the development of discoloration on the skin's surface such as weight gain or loss, environmental toxins, cellular illness, or disease, it can be difficult to protect the skin and prevent dark or light blotches that can appear on the face, hands, neck, chest, etc. Luckily, one effective combatant against discoloration is ginger, and it can be used in two ways to make its benefits that much more effective!

By ingesting ginger, you can provide your body with an abundance of vitamins, minerals, phytochemicals, oils, and enzymes that help support the body's systems and functions that directly affect the skin's health and appearance. Ginger can be used topically, too, as in this Clarifying Mask that provides the skin's surface with antioxidants, amino acids, and toning enzymes and oils that specifically act to rejuvenate the skin's surface with collagen and elastin, helping to promote the regeneration of healthy new skin cells that gradually replace the discolored appearance of scarred skin cells.

TO MAKE 1 APPLICATION OF THE CLARIFYING MASK, USE:

2 tablespoons carrot juice

2 tablespoons apple cider vinegar

1 tablespoon powdered ginger

2 tablespoons honey

1. Combine carrot juice, apple cider vinegar, ginger, and honey in a blender, and blend on medium to high speed for 1–2 minutes, or until all ingredients are thoroughly combined.

2. Apply liberal amounts of the mixture to the face with the fingertips, using a circular motion, focusing on the most problem-prone areas of the skin. Allow mask to remain on the skin for 15–20 minutes.

3. Rinse mask from skin thoroughly using a washcloth soaked with warm water by applying the washcloth to the skin's surface for approximately one minute before using gentle circular motions to cleanse the skin's surface.

Recommendations for use: For best results, this treatment should be used for a time period of 15–20 minutes, 3–7 days per week. Results should be noticeable within 2–4 weeks.

79. PROVIDES RELIEF FOR ITCHY OR SENSITIVE SKIN

Rashes, hives, rosacea, and a number of additional skin conditions result from a disorder or dysfunction that takes place internally. When the body needs to be healed, the tender love and care you provide should focus on the inside *and* the outside. By using a two-step approach with ginger that includes the inclusion of the spicy root in the daily diet as well as topical applications to areas of irritation or inflammation—as seen in the following Healing Mask—anyone can begin a healing process that will free them of itchy, red, sensitive, or inflamed skin. With soothing ingredients that provide relief to the skin, ginger makes an amazing mask that can be used anywhere on the skin, ensuring the skin gets relief and repairing nutrients as the crux of the issue also heals internally. Aromatic, effective, and safe, this ginger Healing Mask can help return your skin to its healthy state without side effects or concerns.

TO MAKE 1 APPLICATION OF THE HEALING MASK, USE:

¼ cup full-fat Greek yogurt

¼ cup coconut oil

1 tablespoon powdered ginger

⅛ teaspoon nutmeg

¼ cup Epsom salts

1. Whisk or blend on medium or high speed until all ingredients are thoroughly combined.
2. Apply the mixture to the skin liberally, focusing on the most problem-prone areas of the skin, then allow mask to remain on the skin for 15–20 minutes.
3. Rinse mask from skin thoroughly using a washcloth soaked with warm water by applying the washcloth to the skin's surface for approximately one minute before using gentle circular motions to cleanse the skin's surface.

Recommendations for use: For best results, this treatment should be used for a time period of 15–20 minutes, 3–7 days per week. Results should be noticeable within 2–4 weeks.

80. SOOTHES SKIN

With ginger's astounding provisions of vitamins, minerals, antioxidants, protein, and collagen- and elastin-building phytochemicals, the all-natural Lotion Bars found in this entry can supply your skin with everything it needs to experience optimal health. These Lotion Bars supply your skin with all-natural ingredients that protect against irritation, inflammation, and illness, and support the regeneration of healthy cells and healthy skin. Maximizing the benefits of these Lotion Bars are the additional phytonutrients of ginger that not only supply medium-chain fatty acids that moisturize and soothe irritated skin, but also minimize irritation, inflammation, and common conditions that can quickly infiltrate and spread within the skin's epidermal layers.

TO MAKE 12 MEDIUM-SIZED SKIN-SOOTHING LOTION BARS, USE:

1 cup coconut oil

1 cup shea or cocoa butter

1 cup beeswax

4 tablespoons powdered ginger

12 drops vitamin E oil

25–50 drops essential oils

1. Combine all ingredients (except vitamin E oil and essential oils) in a 32-ounce glass Mason jar set in a saucepan of heated water for approximately 5–10 minutes, or until ingredients are melted and smooth.

2. Remove the saucepan from heat. Add the essential oils to the mixture, and mix to incorporate well.

3. After combining the ingredients, pour the mixture into molds and set aside to cool and set over 8 hours.

4. Press on the underside of the molds to release the Lotion Bars.

Recommendations for use: For best results, these Lotion Bars should be rubbed on the skin at the end of every bath or shower, or between showers and baths when skin feels dry. Results should be noticeable within 2–4 weeks. Store bars in a cool, dark place for up to 6 months.

81. PROVIDES ANTIOXIDANT SUPPORT TO SKIN

When the body is subjected to toxins, chemicals, and irritants in the environment, food, drinks, etc., one of the first places a reaction appears is on the skin's surface. Luckily, anyone can improve and protect their skin with a supporting, ginger-filled, Antioxidant Scrub that is designed to not only remove toxins from the skin, but also protect against the sun and various cellular changes! With the support of its rich toxin-removing ingredients like antioxidants, vitamins, minerals, enzymes, and oils that promote healing, maintain health, and provide protection, ginger not only adds an aromatic zing to your bath time or shower ritual, but adds essential vitamins and minerals, cell-regenerating support, powerful phytochemicals that speed healing, and potent antioxidants that help stop and reverse cancerous changes. Add to these benefits the moisturizing elements of the yogurt, the antiseptic and antibacterial benefits of the honey, and the antioxidants and stimulation to the skin and bloodstream by the caffeinated coffee, and you have the perfect Antioxidant Scrub that can be used on the skin of the face and body for improvements of the skin's health that are safe, effective, and completely natural!

TO MAKE 1 APPLICATION OF THE ANTIOXIDANT SCRUB, USE:

1 tablespoon ground ginger powder

2 tablespoons finely ground caffeinated coffee beans

1 tablespoon honey

3 tablespoons yogurt

1 tablespoon brown sugar

1. In an 8-ounce Mason jar with a tight-fitting lid, combine all ingredients, then shake the jar vigorously until the contents are thoroughly combined.

2. While showering or bathing, apply the scrub to the skin with a washcloth using circular motions. Rinse, and towel dry as usual.

3. Store remaining scrub in sealed Mason jar in the refrigerator for up to 36–48 hours.

Recommendations for use: For best results, this scrub should be used 5–7 days per week. Results should be noticeable within 2–6 weeks.

82. REDUCES APPEARANCE OF UNDER-EYE CIRCLES, PUFFINESS, AND WRINKLES

The skin under and around the eyes is some of the thinnest and most sensitive, with dark circles, puffiness, and wrinkles appearing there before anywhere else. Lifestyle choices, environmental changes, and nutrient deficiencies have their effects show around the eyes almost immediately. Because this area can be the first to show signs of unhealthy activity within the body, it's absolutely essential to provide nutrients such as skin-regenerating collagen and elastin, as well as protective antioxidants and anti-inflammatory compounds that protect against harmful elements that can cause discoloration, unhealthy cellular changes, inflammation, and irritation. With this homemade Under-Eye Serum, you can use ginger with its plentiful vitamins and minerals, more than fifty potent antioxidants and anti-inflammatory compounds, and unique phytochemical oils like gingerol and shogaol that combine to relieve redness and puffiness, moisturize, calm conditions that lead to dryness and irritation, stimulate circulation, and provide collagen- and elastin-building support for fewer wrinkles. Combine the ginger with effective wrinkle-reducing jojoba oil, rose essential oil, and chamomile essential oil, and you have the perfect beauty regimen addition that can be used day or night, with safe, effective, and quick results.

TO MAKE 5 APPLICATIONS OF THE UNDER-EYE SERUM, USE:

1 ounce jojoba oil
1 ounce fresh ginger juice
5 drops rose essential oil
5 drops chamomile essential oil

1. In a 4–6-oz. glass dropper bottle, combine all oils.
2. To apply, shake dropper well to combine thoroughly. Squeeze a dropper-ful of the oil into the palm of the hand, dip fingertips of the other hand into the solution, and gently apply to the skin around the eyes with circular motions.

Recommendations for use: For best results, this treatment should be used 7 days per week. Results should be noticeable within 1–3 weeks. Store the serum in a cool, dark place. The serum will remain fresh for 2–3 weeks.

83. ENERGIZES SKIN

With all-natural ingredients that not only stimulate the senses and awaken the mind, but also deliver beneficial nutrients to the skin, the following ginger Energizing Spray can supply all the energy you need without harmful chemicals and additives. Enhancing the natural effects of a rejuvenating mist, ginger's unique phytochemicals combine to invigorate the mind, awaken the senses, and energize the body. With unique oils and enzymes that increase thermogenic effects, improve blood flow, and optimize system functioning throughout the body, ginger adds a refreshing and revitalizing spin to a simple spray. Many similar sprays available in specialty shops can cause irritation or dryness on the skin's surface. But this ginger-packed spray is not only safer and less expensive, it also provides natural antioxidants, oils, and moisturizers that can provide protection against harsh elements regularly exposed to the skin, so use it any time you're feeling sluggish!

TO MAKE 1 (8-OUNCE) BOTTLE OF THE ENERGIZING SPRAY, USE:

4 ounces coconut oil

1 ounce almond oil

4 tablespoons grated ginger

10 drops lemon essential oil

10 drops grapefruit essential oil

1. Heat coconut oil and ginger over low heat in a small saucepan for 5–10 minutes, or until fragrant.
2. Remove from heat, add almond oil, and cool. Move cooled mixture to a 16-ounce Mason jar with a tight-fitting lid.
3. Add essential oils, and shake well to combine thoroughly.
4. Move mixture to a spray bottle of your choosing.
5. Spritz the Energizing Spray throughout hair, on face, inside wrists, and over every area of the body, taking care to avoid contact with the eyes.

Recommendations for use: For best results, this spray can be used as often as necessary, 7 days per week. Results should be noticeable immediately upon use. Store spray in a cool, dark room to ensure coconut oil does not harden for future uses, up to 2–3 months.

A LIQUID STATE

If the mixture does harden, place the spray bottle under a stream of warm water or submerge in a large bowl of warm water for 5 minutes, or until mixture returns to a liquid state.

84. REPLENISHES SKIN

Bedtime is the best time for applying a reparative skin cream, mask, or lotion of any kind. While you sleep, the skin absorbs the nutrients of the applied mixture without having to deal with the sweat, chemicals, or other environmental toxins that it's exposed to throughout the day. When you use a gingery Nighttime Body Butter like the one given in this entry, you partake in a repairing, protective, and soothing treatment that not only delivers a plethora of rejuvenating nutrients such as vitamins A, C, and E, and a number of unique enzymes and oils, but also works to protect your skin from those harmful changes that occur during the day.

In addition to ginger's benefits, the aloe vera in this Nighttime Body Butter provides your skin with additional nutrients, antioxidants, and phytochemicals like the proanthocyanidins that intensify the benefits to the skin. And the calming essential oils and soothing moisturizers soften your skin as you're lulled into a deep, restorative sleep. This Nighttime Body Butter makes your skin and your sleep better than you ever dreamed!

TO MAKE 5–10 APPLICATIONS OF THE NIGHTTIME BODY BUTTER, USE:

8 ounces aloe vera gel

3 tablespoons powdered ginger

25–50 drops lavender essential oil

1. In a 12–16-ounce Mason jar with a tight-fitting lid, combine all ingredients.
2. Shake jar to mix well.
3. Apply liberally to any area of skin with the hands, gently massaging the butter into the skin with circular motions, allowing skin to dry before "hitting the sheets."

Recommendations for use: For best results, this treatment should be used 7 nights per week. Results should be noticeable within 1–3 weeks. Store jar in a cool, dark place, for up to one month.

85. REVITALIZES SKIN

There's nothing better than a new soap that makes your skin feel clean and fresh! These ginger-filled Cleansing Bars work to cleanse your skin of topical toxins, removing dirt and grime, opening pores, and allowing for the removal of old, dead skin cells, which promotes the healthy regeneration of new skin cells. These moisturizing, antioxidant-rich Cleansing Bars packed with all-natural ingredients also provide the skin with moisturizing nutrients that nourish the skin's layers and protect them from harsh elements you encounter every single day. And, with the aromatic ingredients like ginger and essential oils, the smell of your skin will be as beautiful as its texture and tone. You'll switch from your old favorite soap and never look back!

TO MAKE 2 CLEANSING BARS, USE:

2½ ounces cocoa butter

1½ ounce shea butter

¾ ounce coconut oil

½ ounce jojoba oil

2 tablespoons ground ginger

1 tablespoon finely ground almonds

2–4 drops lemon essential oil

2–4 drops lavender essential oil

2–4 drops tea tree essential oil

1. Heat butters, coconut and jojoba oils, and ginger over low heat in a small saucepan for 5–10 minutes, or until fragrant.
2. Remove from heat and allow to cool. Move cooled mixture to a 12–16-ounce Mason jar with a tight-fitting lid.
3. Stir in powdered ginger and ground almonds, along with essential oils.
4. Pour into molds and allow to set for 8 hours. Once the bars are solid and firm, pop the bars out of the mold and wrap individually in plastic wrap.
5. To cleanse the skin of the face and body, wet a Cleansing Bar with warm water, scrub to soften the bar, and massage the melted oils from the bar into the skin. Rinse with a warm, damp washcloth.

Recommendations for use: For best results, this bar should be used 5–7 days per week. Results should be noticeable within 1–3 uses. Store bars in a cool, dark place for up to 1 month.

86. EXFOLIATES AND MOISTURIZES LIPS

One of the first things people notice about the face are the lips, and this essential part of the face helps us eat, drink, speak, and formulate perfect facial expressions for every occasion! When the lips are constantly exposed to the elements, moving from wet to dry conditions, and being smothered with saliva, foods, and liquids, they can easily become red, dry, irritated, cracked, inflamed, and even infected. Fortunately, ginger is able to improve lip health naturally! The lip-saving combination of the all-natural ingredients included in this following exfoliating recipe use ginger's awesome benefits to not only provide your lips with the essential vitamins, minerals, antioxidants, and phytochemicals that protect and revive your skin, but also promote the healthy regeneration of collagen and elastin and ensure healthy circulation to the area. This simple sugar-packed Lip-Smoothing Exfoliate will leave you with perfect lips . . . with which to kiss your dull, cracked lips of the past goodbye!

TO MAKE 20 APPLICATIONS OF THE LIP-SMOOTHING EXFOLIATE, USE:

1 tablespoon ginger oil

¼ cup coconut oil

2 tablespoons granulated sugar

1. In an 8-ounce Mason jar with a tight-fitting lid, combine ingredients and shake well to combine thoroughly.
2. Apply the mixture to the lips, gently scrubbing the lips with the fingers using circular massaging motions for 2–3 minutes.
3. Rinse the mixture from the lips using warm water.

Recommendations for use: For best results, this treatment can be used daily. Results should be noticeable within 1–2 applications. Store the remaining treatment in a cool, dark place (such as a cabinet) for up to one month.

Chapter 4

HAIR CARE

The exposure to the variety of damaging routines your hair likely endures is pretty alarming, when you think about it. Between unprotected exposure to sunlight, chemicals in your hair-care products, toxins in the environment, and the heat and stress you may apply to those strands every day through the styling processes, it's no wonder that hair becomes dull, dry, and unmanageable. In an effort to improve the health, quality, and appearance of your hair, you may be tempted to purchase and apply those new products on the shelves in the beauty aisle that promise to restore health and beauty to your locks, but those promises may fall flat, leaving your hair lackluster and even more damaged than before.

So, save your hair and your wallet from the latest fads in hair care, and opt for do-it-yourself products that include ginger, which can help repair, revitalize, and restore shine and beauty to every strand of your hair safely and effectively. By combining powdered, juiced, or grated ginger with additional specific ingredients that naturally intensify the benefits to your hair, you can achieve beautiful, healthier looking hair in just a few simple treatments! Enjoy!

THE HAIR'S HEALTH

The same nutrients that help hair health get a miraculous boost when the addition of ginger is used in hair applications. With elastin-encouraging oils and enzymes that help hair strands become stronger, combined with the natural vitamins and minerals that promote healthy hair growth, ginger can be used in a variety of do-it-yourself homemade hair tonics and treatments that can improve the health of your hair naturally!

87. STIMULATES HAIR GROWTH

Long, luxurious, healthy hair has been one of the most sought-after physical attributes in almost every culture in history, and that beautiful "accessory" is still the highlight of many women's beauty today. With hair extensions, expensive treatments, and formulas promising to deliver long locks of beauty to any woman with time and money, it's easy to understand why many women seek out safer, more natural, less expensive methods to achieve the long hair of their dreams. Ginger naturally encourages proper blood circulation, can provide the scalp with relieving moisturizers to optimize scalp health, and promotes the health of strands with rich protective and preventative oils and enzymes. With this combination of ginger and jojoba oil, a staple of Native American culture, any woman can achieve full locks of hair that are not only long, but healthier and more beautiful than ever before, too!

TO MAKE 2–4 TREATMENTS OF THE GROWTH TREATMENT, USE:

1 cup coconut oil

1 cup jojoba oil

4 tablespoons powdered ginger

10–20 drops of lavender essential oil

1. In a 20-ounce glass Mason jar with a tight-fitting lid, combine all ingredients and shake well to combine thoroughly.
2. Wet hair thoroughly and towel dry to remove excess moisture.
3. Soak hair with the mixture, massaging into the scalp and combing through strands to ensure even distribution throughout.
4. Cover hair with plastic wrap, which allows your body heat to warm the treatment naturally. Allow the treatment to set on hair for 30 minutes before rinsing thoroughly.
5. Towel dry and style as usual.

Recommendations for use: For best results, this treatment should be used once or twice weekly. Results should be noticeable within 4–8 weeks. Store the remaining treatment in a cool, dark place (such as a cabinet) for up to one month.

88. IMPROVES DRY, BRITTLE, AND DAMAGED HAIR

Dry, brittle hair can be a tough issue to tangle with. Whether the condition is due to chlorine, water conditions, extensive styling treatments, or genetics, transforming your hair from dry and damaged to soft and luxurious can be as simple as adding all-natural, reparative ingredients like ginger to your hair's beauty regimen. With the simple combination of nutrient-rich aloe vera, clarifying apple cider vinegar, moisturizing almond oil, and antioxidant- and oil-rich ginger, this homemade mixture of naturally restorative ingredients will revive and rejuvenate every strand, while nourishing the scalp and the roots to ensure the health of future growth, as well. Through clarifying toxins, moisturizing, and delivering the very nutrients your hair needs to remain healthy, strong, and moisturized, with ginger you can say goodbye to those dry, brittle locks forever!

1. In a 12–16-ounce glass Mason jar with a tight-fitting lid, combine ingredients and shake well to combine thoroughly.
2. Wet hair thoroughly and towel dry to remove excess water.
3. Soak hair with the mixture, massaging into the scalp and combing through strands to ensure even distribution throughout.
4. Cover hair with plastic wrap, which allows your body heat to warm the treatment naturally. Allow the treatment to set on hair for 20–30 minutes before rinsing thoroughly.
5. Towel dry and style as usual.

Recommendations for use: For best results, this treatment should be used once or twice weekly. Results should be noticeable within 4–8 weeks. Store the remaining treatment in a cool, dark place (such as a cabinet) for up to one month.

TO MAKE 2 APPLICATIONS OF THE DRY HAIR TREATMENT, USE:

2 tablespoons powdered ginger

½ cup aloe vera

¼ cup apple cider vinegar

¼ cup almond oil

89. TREATS DANDRUFF

Dandruff is one of the most difficult hair conditions to deal with. Categorized by unsightly white flakes that shake from a dry, itchy scalp, anyone suffering from dandruff knows how uncomfortable and embarrassing it can be. While a number of products on the market promise to deliver relief from dandruff, many of them may further exacerbate the very source of the dandruff by drying out the scalp and causing even more irritation. For a simple do-it-yourself conditioning treatment that will provide your scalp with the nutrition and moisture it needs to prevent dryness, irritation, and inflammation in the future, look no further than ginger! This root's powerful pH-restoring, anti-inflammatory, and anti-septic benefits combine with cleansing tea tree oil, clarifying lemon juice, and conditioning coconut oil to naturally banish dandruff flakes while improving the look, feel, and condition of your hair, safely and effectively!

TO MAKE 1–2 APPLICATIONS OF THE DANDRUFF TREATMENT, USE:

2 tablespoons ginger juice

2 tablespoons powdered ginger

20 drops tea tree oil

2 tablespoons lemon juice

½ cup coconut oil

1. In a 12–16-ounce glass Mason jar with a tight-fitting lid, combine ingredients and use an immersion blender to combine thoroughly.
2. Wet hair thoroughly and towel dry to remove excess water.
3. Apply the mixture to the scalp, massaging into the scalp and combing through strands to ensure even distribution throughout.
4. Cover hair with plastic wrap, which allows your body heat to warm the treatment naturally. Allow the treatment to set on hair for 15–20 minutes before rinsing thoroughly.
5. Towel dry and style as usual.

Recommendations for use: For best results, this treatment should be used once or twice weekly. Results should be noticeable within 1–2 weeks. Store the remaining treatment in a cool, dark place (such as a cabinet) for up to one month.

90. SMOOTHS SPLIT ENDS

All hair seems to fall victim to unsightly split ends at one time or another. Fortunately, a simple combination of all-natural ingredients—including the trusty ginger root—can deliver nutrients and soothing reparative phytochemicals that naturally restore your hair's health and minimize the split-end scenario. Combined with coconut, almond, and olive oil, along with a ripe avocado, ginger's moisturizing and protective benefits that come from its rich stores of nourishing vitamins A, C, and E not only improve your hair's health, but keep every strand protected from the elements, treatments, and conditions like excessive sun exposure, heat treatments, and chemicals used for styling that contributed to split ends in the past!

1. In a bowl, mash avocado with a fork or immersion blender, and combine all ingredients thoroughly.
2. Move mixture to a 16-ounce Mason jar with a tight-fitting lid, or a container suitable for storage and easy use.
3. Coat your slightly dampened hair's ends with the mixture, working the treatment up throughout the hair and massaging the mixture into the scalp.
4. Allow the treatment to set on hair for 20–30 minutes, covered with plastic wrap or a shower cap before rinsing thoroughly.
5. Towel dry and style as usual.

Recommendations for use: For best results, this treatment should be used 2–4 days per week. Results should be noticeable within 2–4 weeks.

TO MAKE 1–2 APPLICATIONS OF THE SPLIT-END TREATMENT, USE:

1 ripe avocado, seed and skin removed

2 tablespoons ginger juice

1 tablespoon powdered ginger

⅛ cup coconut oil

⅛ cup almond oil

⅛ cup jojoba oil

91. CONDITIONS COLOR-TREATED HAIR

Color-treated hair is exposed to a number of harsh ingredients and methods that can strip moisture and nutrients from your scalp and strands in the process of color change. The good news is, through the use of ginger, the dry, damaged locks left behind by hair color can stop today. Long used for its moisturizing benefits, ginger is able to join forces with the naturally nutrient-restoring medium-chain fatty acid–packed coconut oil and aloe vera that both help nutrients penetrate the layers of protein in the hair shaft. Added to this healthy trio are the clarifying and moisturizing honey and lemon juice that rid the hair of toxins and buildup while restoring much-needed, hair-healthy moisture to the color-treated locks in need. Natural, effective, and completely safe, this combination is a hair-healthy recipe for color-treated locks that need a little love.

1. In a 12–16-ounce glass Mason jar with a tight-fitting lid, combine ingredients and use an immersion blender to combine ingredients thoroughly.
2. Wet hair thoroughly and towel dry to remove excess moisture.
3. Soak hair with the mixture, massaging into the scalp and combing through strands to ensure even distribution throughout.
4. Cover hair with plastic wrap, which allows your body heat to warm the treatment naturally. Allow the treatment to set on hair for 20–30 minutes before rinsing thoroughly.
5. Towel dry and style as usual.

Recommendations for use: For best results, this treatment should be used once or twice weekly. Results should be noticeable within 2–4 weeks. Store the remaining treatment in a cool, dark place (such as a cabinet) for 2–3 weeks.

TO MAKE 1–2 APPLICATIONS OF THE CONDITIONING MASK, USE:

2 tablespoons powdered ginger

½ cup coconut oil

½ cup aloe vera juice

2 tablespoons honey

1 tablespoon lemon juice

92. CONDITIONS NON-COLOR-TREATED HAIR

Conditioner is an amazing product! With nutrients, proteins, and plenty of smoothing elements that combine to promote the healthy growth of hair, the natural moisturizers and conditioners also act to protect the strand shafts against damage while creating a smooth appearance and feel to the hair. To avoid dry, dull tangles, and the plastic-packed synthetic conditioners found in most stores, you can opt for an all-natural leave-in conditioning treatment that clarifies the strands of toxins and buildup, and delivers intense moisture and nutrients that help you achieve a beautiful, lightweight, clean, conditioned head of hair that not only looks great, but feels great, too!

Ginger provides natural conditioning benefits that not only help improve the look and feel of hair, but also improve hair's health. Ginger's two naturally occurring unique oils, gingerol and shogaol, double as powerful antioxidants that help protect hair against damage from environmental conditions like heat and pollution while also protecting against damage within the cells and strands of hair. With the simple addition of ginger, anyone can achieve naturally protected and conditioned hair that is healthy and vibrant on the inside and out!

TO MAKE 1 APPLICATION OF THE LEAVE-IN CONDITIONER, USE:

1 cup water
½ cup aloe vera juice
3 tablespoons ginger juice
1 tablespoon apple cider vinegar

1. In a spray bottle, combine all ingredients and shake vigorously to combine thoroughly.
2. After shampooing and rinsing hair, apply the mixture to the scalp and strands, massaging the scalp and combing through the hair to coat strands evenly.
3. Towel dry and style as usual.

Recommendations for use: For best results, this treatment should be used 5–7 days per week. Results should be noticeable within 1–3 uses.

93. CREATES NATURAL HIGHLIGHTS IN HAIR

With enough damage being bestowed by the chemicals and styling processes required for highlights, the smartest way to avoid excessively color-treating hair, or causing damage from excessive treatments, is to turn to all-natural combinations of healing, nutrient-rich ingredients that not only repair and protect hair from dryness and damage, but also lighten the locks! This simple Lightening Treatment uses natural unique oils and a number of powerful phytochemicals found in the ginger root that enhance the lightening process effectively and safeguard the hair against damage. Through the use of this treatment, you can enjoy highlighted hair that retains its health, moisture, and shine without concern of dryness, damage, or disastrous outcomes.

TO MAKE 1–2 APPLICATIONS OF THE LIGHTENING TREATMENT, USE:

2 tablespoons powdered ginger

1 tablespoon ginger juice

1 cup apple cider vinegar

¾ cup raw honey

1. In a 16-ounce glass Mason jar with a tight-fitting lid, combine ingredients and blend using an immersion blender to combine thoroughly.
2. Soak hair with the mixture, massaging into the scalp and combing through strands to ensure even distribution throughout.
3. Cover hair with plastic wrap, which allows your body heat to warm the treatment naturally. Allow the treatment to set on hair for 4–6 hours, before rinsing thoroughly.
4. Towel dry and style as usual.

Recommendations for use: For best results, this treatment should be used once or twice weekly. Results should be noticeable within 1–2 applications. Any remaining treatment should be stored in a cool, dark place for up to 2 weeks.

94. TAMES FRIZZ

Striking straight, curly, or wavy hair, it only takes a hint of humidity for frizz to take over. Fortunately, the all-natural ingredients like ginger, jojoba oil, and aloe vera that provide your hair with a calming combination of oils, moisturizers, and nutrients can calm frizz without turning strands oily or coated with residue. A frizz-taming treatment like the serum found here can be used as often as necessary, and without the risk of any harsh side effects, excessive dryness, or damage to the hair. Add the beautiful aroma to the safe, effective, all-natural benefits of this beautifying treatment, and this do-it-yourself frizz-fighting potion will take the place of any other product in just one use!

2. Add powdered ginger and ground almonds, along with essential oils. Shake to combine.

3. Spray mixture lightly on problem areas of the hair, brushing the treatment through the strands. While applying, take care to avoid saturating the hair or applying the mixture to the scalp, to avoid over-treating and developing an oily or greasy appearance.

Recommendations for use: For best results, this treatment should be used as often as necessary. Results should be noticeable immediately. Remaining treatment should be stored in a cool, dark place for up to 3–4 weeks.

TO MAKE 2–4 APPLICATIONS OF THE FRIZZ-TAMING SERUM, USE:

2 tablespoons ginger oil

1 cup water

½ cup jojoba oil

½ cup aloe vera juice

1 tablespoon powdered ginger

1 tablespoon ground almonds

10 drops essential oil of your choosing

1. In a spray bottle, combine ginger oil, water, jojoba oil, and aloe vera juice.

95. PROTECTS HAIR FROM HEAT DAMAGE

The use of heat during the daily styling processes engaged in by millions of women may create a beautiful look, but can cause damage that dulls, dries out, and delays healthy hair growth. While many of the products designed to protect hair from heat damage may promise to protect and repair, few deliver the intense moisture and protection needed by excessively heat-treated hair. The all-natural Heat Damage Serum found in this entry features ingredients like antioxidant-rich and protective ginger oil that will help repair damaged strands and rejuvenate the scalp for healthy hair growth, as well as potassium-rich banana that acts as a moisturizing protectant to combat heat damage inside the hair strands as well as on the outside, and moisture-restoring honey that gives hair bounce, shine, and health. With the addition of protective olive and almond oils that also contribute essential proteins to protect against breakage, this collagen- and elastin-promoting serum will not only help to protect against heat damage, but will your return your damaged strands to the beautiful, luxurious locks they once were!

TO MAKE 1 APPLICATION OF THE HEAT DAMAGE SERUM, USE:

2 tablespoons ginger oil
1 ripe banana, peeled
2 tablespoons aloe vera juice
1 tablespoon jojoba oil

1. In a 16-ounce glass Mason jar with a tight-fitting lid, combine ingredients and use an immersion blender to combine thoroughly.
2. Wet hair thoroughly and towel dry to remove excess moisture.
3. Apply mixture to hair, massaging into the scalp and combing through strands to ensure even distribution throughout.
4. Cover hair with plastic wrap, which allows your body heat to warm the treatment naturally. Allow the treatment to set on hair for 20–30 minutes before rinsing thoroughly.
5. Towel dry and style as usual.

Recommendations for use: For best results, this treatment should be used once or twice weekly. Results should be noticeable within 4–8 weeks.

96. CLEANSES AND MOISTURIZES HAIR AS A DRY SHAMPOO

Able to deliver nutrients, remove oil, and cleanse strands of buildup, dry shampoo can be used by anyone on the go, or in need of a quick refresh . . . without the trouble of a time-consuming shower, wash, and style. The issues for some who use dry shampoos quickly became apparent, though. As a result of the chemical cleansers, moisturizers, and drying elements contained in each treatment, the dry shampoo can make some hair types either excessively dry, oily, or otherwise undesirable.

Ginger and the other ingredients in the Dry Shampoo recipe found in this entry combine to provide nutrients, light unique oils, and protein-rich collagen- and elastin-production promoting phytochemicals to your hair, which means that this dry shampoo can be used regardless of hair type, length, or condition. Health-promoting, beauty-boosting, safe, effective, and all-natural, this dry shampoo is the best thing you could give your hair when it's in need of something, but you have time for nothing!

TO MAKE 1–3 APPLICATIONS OF THE DRY SHAMPOO, USE:

2 tablespoons powdered ginger

½ cup organic cornstarch

10 drops lavender essential oil (optional)

1. In an 8–12-ounce glass Mason jar with a tight-fitting lid, combine all ingredients and shake well to combine thoroughly.
2. Apply the mixture to the hair, starting at the scalp and combing through the strands.
3. Use application as often as necessary, rinsing and washing hair normally when needed.

Recommendations for use: For best results, this dry shampoo can be used 5–7 days per week. Results should be noticeable immediately. Any remaining treatments should be stored in a cool, dark place for up to 6 months.

97. IMPROVES HAIR'S SHINE

Shine, shimmer, luminosity! These three words capture one of the most desirable characteristics of healthy hair. With strands that reflect light perfectly, capture the sun's radiance in every shadow and shine, and don't project a single moment of dullness, shiny hair is the personification of health. People associate shiny hair with health because hair requires nutrition and care in order to be shiny.

Luckily, using ginger, you can simply and easily create a shine-improving spray for your hair in no time. In this simple concoction, ginger stars as the main ingredient and contributes unique oils, nutrients, proteins, antioxidants, and moisturizers that not only help to deliver healthy essentials to the hair, but help to protect the hair against damage that can strip strands of their health and shine. In addition to ginger, the jojoba, olive, and vitamin E oils improve the look and feel of the hair by contributing moisturizers and carrier enzymes that help those moisturizers penetrate deep within the strands where they're most needed.

TO MAKE 5–10 APPLICATIONS OF THE SHINE SPRAY, USE:

2 tablespoons ginger oil

¼ cup jojoba oil

¼ cup olive oil

¼ vitamin E oil

½ cup aloe vera juice

1. In a spray bottle, combine ingredients and shake well to combine thoroughly.
2. Wet hair thoroughly and towel dry to remove excess moisture.
3. Spray hair with the mixture liberally, massaging into the scalp and combing through strands to ensure even distribution throughout.
4. Towel dry to remove excess if necessary, and style as usual.

Recommendations for use: For best results, this treatment can be used daily, and results should be noticeable immediately. Store the spray bottle in a cool, dark place (such as a cabinet) for up to 6 months.

98. MOISTURIZES AND PROTECTS HAIR

Hair masks are designed to infuse your hair with a variety of beneficial nutrients, but a homemade hair mask including ginger and all of its plentiful antioxidants, vitamins, minerals, oils, and enzymes works to restore moisture, repair with proteins, encourage strength and growth with collagen and elastin, and protect against damage that can occur from daily styling, products, and even exposure to the elements. The ginger oil found in this intense Moisturizing Mask recipe works hand in hand with the honey, aloe vera, and jojoba and almond oils to provide all of the essentials the hair needs, including a plethora of phytochemicals that moisturize deep into the scalp and beyond the hair shaft of every strand, to provide your locks with luscious moisture!

TO MAKE 1–2 APPLICATIONS OF THE MOISTURIZING MASK, USE:

2 tablespoons ginger oil

¼ cup raw honey

¼ cup aloe vera juice

¼ cup jojoba oil

¼ cup almond oil

1. In a 16-ounce glass Mason jar with a tight-fitting lid, combine ingredients and use an immersion blender to combine thoroughly.
2. Wet hair thoroughly and towel dry to remove excess moisture.
3. Soak hair with the mixture, massaging into the scalp and combing through strands to ensure even distribution throughout.
4. Cover hair with plastic wrap, which allows your body heat to warm the treatment naturally. Allow the treatment to set on hair for 30 minutes before rinsing thoroughly.
5. Towel dry and style as usual.

Recommendations for use: For best results, this treatment should be used once or twice weekly. Results should be noticeable within 1–2 applications. Any excess mixture remaining after the application should be stored in a cool, dry place for up to 2 weeks.

99. ADDS VOLUME TO HAIR

With countless products on the market claiming to improve the volume of your hair, it can be confusing to choose the one that will benefit your hair type and your hair's needs. While these products make claims and guarantees that promise to deliver the perfect head of hair you desire, the results often fall flat. Adding to the less-than-desirable results is the possibility of damage to the scalp and strands from the alcohol and synthetic additives that are commonly found in volumizing shampoos, conditioners, and treatments that can leave your hair frizzy, greasy, and lackluster. Luckily, there is an all-natural alternative that you can quickly create in your own home and apply in just minutes that delivers real results.

By combining ginger powder, apple cider vinegar, and lemon juice, you can create a volumizing rinse that helps you achieve the look you desire by cleansing the scalp and strands of the grime and residue that weigh hair down, resulting in little to no volume. Helping nurture the scalp with antioxidants and enzymes of all three ingredients, this solution not only adds volume, but promotes hair health, too!

TO MAKE 1 APPLICATION OF THE HAIR VOLUMIZING TREATMENT, USE:

1 tablespoon powdered ginger
1 teaspoon lemon juice
¼ cup apple cider vinegar
½ cup cool water

1. In a 16-ounce glass Mason jar with a tight-fitting lid, combine ingredients and shake vigorously to combine thoroughly.
2. Shower, shampoo, and condition as usual, and apply solution to scalp and throughout strands to saturate.
3. Allow solution to set for 2–4 minutes before rinsing thoroughly.
4. Towel dry and style as usual.

Recommendations for use: For best results, this treatment should be used 2–3 times weekly. Results should be noticeable within 1–2 applications. Any remaining mixture should be stored in a cool, dark place for up to 5–7 days.

100. CLARIFIES HAIR

To stay healthy, hair requires nutrients from our diet, moisture from conditioners, and cleansing, clarifying benefits from shampoos and cleansers that remove dirt, grime, and toxins from the hair. With all these requirements, it's easy to see how daily hair-care routines can be interrupted by a busy daily schedule. When a hair-care regimen gets placed on hold, the result can be oily, greasy, and residue-coated hair. This Hair Clarifying Treatment combines the amazing antimicrobial and antiseptic ginger with cleansing lemon juice and apple cider vinegar, and moisturizing ingredients like aloe and honey that not only keep the hair and scalp clear, but do so with health benefits that care for hair long into the future! With this safe, effective treatment that can cleanse strands of impurities and resist the buildup of residue, your hair will be healthy in no time!

TO MAKE 1–2 APPLICATIONS OF THE HAIR CLARIFYING TREATMENT, USE:

2 tablespoons ginger oil

1 tablespoon lemon juice

¼ cup apple cider vinegar

½ cup aloe vera juice

¼ cup honey

1. In a 16-ounce glass Mason jar with a tight-fitting lid, combine ingredients and use an immersion blender to combine thoroughly.
2. Wet hair thoroughly and towel dry to remove excess moisture.
3. Soak hair with the mixture, massaging into the scalp and combing through strands to ensure even distribution throughout.
4. Cover hair with plastic wrap, which allows your body heat to warm the treatment naturally. Allow the treatment to set on hair for 15–20 minutes before rinsing thoroughly.
5. Towel dry and style as usual.

Recommendations for use: For best results, this treatment should be used once or twice weekly. Results should be noticeable within 1–2 applications. Any remaining mixture should be stored in a cool, dark place for up to 5–7 days.

INDEX

ABOUT THE AUTHOR

Britt Brandon is a Certified Personal Trainer and Certified Fitness Nutrition Specialist (certified by the International Sports Science Association, ISSA) and Health Coach (certified by the American Council on Exercise, ACE) who has enjoyed writing books that focus on clean eating, fitness, and unique health-promoting ingredients such as apple cider vinegar, coconut oil, and aloe vera for Adams Media. In her time with Adams, she has published eleven books, including *The Everything® Green Smoothies Book, The Everything® Eating Clean Cookbook, What Color Is Your Smoothie?, The Everything® Eating Clean Cookbook for Vegetarians, The Everything® Healthy Green Drinks Book, The Everything® Guide to Pregnancy Nutrition & Health, Apple Cider Vinegar for Health,* and *Coconut Oil for Health.* As a competitive athlete, trainer, mom of three small children, and fitness and nutrition blogger on her own website (*www.ultimatefitmom.com*), she is well versed in the holistic approaches to keeping one's self in top performing condition . . . and actually uses ginger daily in food and drinks, as well as in many home remedies.